56751

231.73
MEL

John's College
Library
te for return

D1381063

York St John C...
Fountains Learning Centre

Please return this item on or before the date
stamped below

- 5 FEB 2004	1 3 JAN 2006	2 6 MAY 2006
	RETURNED	
- 1 APR 2004	0 6 JUN 2007	RETURNED
- 2 JUN 2004	RETURNED	1 6 MAY 2008
	1 8 MAY 2011	
RETURNED		
- 2 FEB 2007		

Fines are payable for late return

CANCELLED

WITHDRAWN

17 JUN 2022

Coll. of Ripon & York St John

3 8025 00163522 9

HEALING MIRACLES

HEALING
MIRACLES

An Examination from History and Experience
of the Place of Miracle
in Christian Thought and Medical Practice

M. A. H. MELINSKY

Vicar of St. Stephen's Church, Norwich
Chaplain to the Norfolk and Norwich Hospital
Director of the Norwich Branch of the Samaritans

THE LIBRARY
COLLEGE OF RIPON AND YORK ST. JOHN
COLLEGE ROAD, RIPON HG

LONDON
A. R. MOWBRAY & CO LTD

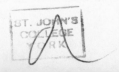
ST. JOHN'S
COLLEGE
YORK

© A. R. Mowbray & Co Ltd 1968
Printed in Great Britain by
Alden & Mowbray Ltd at the Alden Press, Oxford
SBN 264 65562 1
First published in 1968

ST. JOHN'S COLLEGE, YORK.

CLASS D	ACCESSION No
231/73	36682
CHECKED	DATE
	10-6-70

Dedicated to
two sustainers of the dialogue
between religion and science,
both my teachers at Cambridge,
Charles E. Raven, formerly Master,
and Ian T. Ramsey, formerly Fellow and Chaplain,
of Christ's College,
with respect, affection, and gratitude

Forewords

BY THE RIGHT REVEREND IAN T. RAMSEY, DD
Bishop of Durham

WHEN I took the topic of Miracles as the subject of my Inaugural Lecture at Oxford, I did so because it seemed to me that on this topic was focused a whole range of converging and controversial issues. Mr Melinsky's book is especially valuable for the way in which it discusses miracles in this wide setting, placing them squarely in their biblical background, and showing their changing place in Christian thought and apologetic. He brings to bear on his discussion contemporary insights in the philosophy of religion, and shows how biblical and scientific criticism influences our understanding of miracles.

But Mr Melinsky's wide survey does not stop even here. He then concentrates on healing miracles as a salient topic on the frontier between religion and medicine, and this leads him to discuss the changing relations of medicine and theology down the years from the origins of modern medicine in ancient Greece.

Mr Melinsky shirks no difficulty whether the intellectual one of grappling with the alleged miraculous element of a cure, or the pastoral one of ministering to those in hospital, who might, on a wrong view of miracle, have wrong expectations about God's healing power.

This is not only a book for discussion between clergy and doctors, but a book which will help all Christian believers to grapple successfully with one of the toughest areas of their belief. No topic more than that of miracle needs the broad perspective, the thoroughness, the frankness, the fair-mindedness and the balanced judgment which Mr Melinsky displays.

I am very glad to commend this book by my former pupil, which shows so well how, in the ministry of a priest, there can be profitably united sound learning and a deep pastoral concern.

BY DR R. A. LAMBOURNE, BD, MB, ChB, DPM
Lecturer in Pastoral Studies, University of Birmingham

A QUICK comparison of current medical journals with those of twenty years ago will demonstrate that in the interim medicine has become much more self-conscious and self-critical whilst it has become increasingly involved professionally in a whole range of social, moral and political decisions which in the previous years were considered matters purely of private interest and conscience. For example the staggering successes of modern medicine have produced a rush of new personal ethical decisions concerning such matters as the artificial prolongation of life, genetic planning, transplant donation and the use of psychedelic drugs, to name but a few. Even more important has been the realisation that good medicine must be worldly medicine. This is epitomised by the shock of discovering that famine and political revolution may follow the success of humane medicine in prolonging life and thus producing a population explosion. It is no longer possible to keep medicine and political planning in separate compartments, and least of all in that very area which at first glance might appear to be most scientific, namely medical research! The clinician finds himself willy-nilly engaged in applied political and moral science. The implications of this for the style of life of medicine and thus for medical education obviously requires profound thought.

This book on miracles will assist such profound thought since the author is requiring us to take a fresh look at the Christian origins of one of the main sources of that medical humanism which, mostly unconsciously, shapes the very details of our twentieth-century western medicine. The author's examination of the Gospels reminds us that this source was concerned with healing within a total human concept. The miracles cannot even begin to be understood except within the whole plan of God for the totality of matter and especially within his plan for the health and wholeness of all nations. The author demolishes the popular view that the miracles are to be contrasted with modern medicine by virtue of supposed magical–supernatural content, and insists by contrast that both are to be judged according to their rationality. Moreover the test of rationality is a very pragmatic one. Do they define and effect the real health of whole people and whole nations according to the vision of healthy man given to those who experienced the life of Christ? By this practical test some of our programmes of medical research and clinical practice may compare unfavourably with Christ's healing work because they too widely miss the mark set by the needs of millions of medically underprivileged people!

Any serious study of the healing miracles goes to the heart of medicine because it must examine the philosophy of science and also the measure of health. This book does this and so makes us simultaneously look at contemporary medicine and the Gospels. By doing so it paves the way for radical decisions about both God and the structures of medicine and medical education. For this reason it can be commended to all doctors who love their work and wish to see that neither time nor effort is wasted in bringing health and wholeness to all peoples. Because medicine concerns us all, laymen will be equally interested. Canon Melinsky writes sensitively from long experience of men and women patients he has known as a Hospital Chaplain. I hope this book has the success he deserves.

Preface

THE substance of this book was first given as five Lent Lectures in Norwich Cathedral in 1967. I should like to record my appreciation to the Dean and Chapter for the honour of this invitation, and also to my audience for their attention to over-long lectures and for their contribution in discussion afterwards. The original content of these lectures is here considerably revised and expanded.

I am glad of the opportunity to express my thanks to three people who have offered much helpful guidance and criticism: to the Rt Revd I. T. Ramsey, Bishop of Durham, who has advised me on the theological and philosophical side; to Dr G. H. Day who has saved me from many medical blunders, as also from many infelicities of expression; and to Canon W. Purcell, Literary Adviser to the publishers, who has taken a keen interest in the project from its birth. For my interpretations and conclusions they are in no way responsible.

The writing of this book was only made possible by several short stays at the Community of All Hallows at Ditchingham, whose tranquil atmosphere is always an inspiration. To the Mother Superior and to Sister Kathleen at the guest-house my sincere thanks.

I am happy to acknowledge a deep debt of gratitude to Mrs M. van Rijn who has toiled ungrudgingly with the typing and re-typing of my manuscript; and also to Dr Day and the Revd A. A. Coldwells for much laborious care in proof-reading.

This book carries two Forewords, one by the Bishop of

Durham and one by Dr R. A. Lambourne, whose companionship in the Institute of Religion and Medicine has been a constant encouragement. My hope in writing it is that it may in some small measure forward the objects of this Institute which are 'to seek greater knowledge of the principles on which health in its widest spiritual, mental, and physical sense is based, and to promote a better understanding and co-operation between all people who are engaged in the fields of religion and medicine'.

M.A.H.M.

Norwich,
St Luke's Day 1967

Contents

of genius in England 1650–1720. Abroad Petit, Buffon, Lamarck, Pasteur. Neglect of mental illness until Pinel. Mesmer and Charcot. Freud and the unconscious. Assessment of psychoanalysis as a theory of meaning.

Psychosomatic or whole-man approach to illness. Examples from ailments of heart, stomach, colon; tuberculosis; asthma; skin; eye; rheumatism; bone. Cancer. Inadequacy of old mechanistic models of nature.

The approach of the Form Critics examined. Miracles in St Mark (with parallels from other Gospels); in 'Q' (i.e. St Luke and St Matthew in parallel); in St Matthew only; in St Luke only; in St John.

Recapitulation of argument. Difficulty of analysing miraculous element in a cure illustrated by an example. The claims of Lourdes examined. Remythologising the miracles in terms of community care for the whole person.

The problem of suffering. Connexion of sickness with sin. Sin as despair. Sin as distorted relationships. Love as the Christian treatment. Prayer for the sick. Sacrament and miracle. Conclusion.

NOTE

The two-figure references in the text are to books listed in the Bibliography on pages 179–183. The first figure, in italics, refers to the book there numbered, and the second figure to the page of that book. The letter 'f' following a number refers the reader to pages (or in the case of the Bible to chapters or verses) following that cited.

HEALING MIRACLES

1. Definition of Terms

WHOEVER sets sail to explore the subject of miracle risks shipwreck on a variety of shoals. He must face major difficulties of theology, philosophy, history, and science, and must call in question assumptions lying behind these various disciplines which have long lain unexamined.

In the modern world of specialised study and disciplinary isolation he is a bold man who tries to link together into some sort of pattern the various aspects of miracle which touch on these varied fields. Little major work on miracles in their broader aspect has been produced in this country for a generation. Recently in one of the oldest and most renowned cathedral cities of England a request was made to the clergy by schoolteachers for a lecture on the subject of miracles, and no volunteer from the whole diocese could be found.

It follows that much of what is written in this book leans heavily on the work of experts in several different fields. In addition it was put together in the course of a busy pastoral ministry with little leisure for the delights of scholarship. But it was a hospital ministry which forced upon me a reconsideration of many assumptions, because the scientific medical approach to sick people is by itself obviously inadequate. Further, the medical world is beginning a radical re-thinking of some of its own basic categories, and this has not made the present task easier.

A hundred years ago most Christians would have argued that the existence of miracle stories in the gospels proved that Christ was divine. Today a great number of people argue that the existence of miracle stories in the gospels proves that the gospels are unreliable—so unreliable that their fundamental claims can safely be ignored. Each of these attitudes is based on a complex of presuppositions which is seldom brought into the light of day. If each is carefully examined it will go far to cut a way through a jungle of confusion and misunderstanding.

The concept of miracle in Christian thought is grounded in the Bible, and more particularly in the New Testament, and so our definition must start there. Inspection will show that a miracle is not a simple but a complex event, with two major features. First an event is claimed to have happened which does not conform with the normal run of human experience. This is a source of wonder (which is the basic meaning of the word 'miracle'). But, second, in and through this event a claim is made for a particular disclosure of God, his power, his activity, indeed his concern and love. In this respect a miracle is also a sign (Greek—*sēmeion*) which is a common description of it in the New Testament.

Miracle stories can be graded according to the degree of non-conformity involved, but this is neither very precise nor very helpful. At the most extreme is a radical non-conformity, like the sun going backwards. In the middle are acts of healing, which have natural counterparts, but in different ways. The least remarkable are miracles of co-incidence, as for example most of the plagues in Egypt, where it is generally assumed that the plagues are natural occurrences, but their miraculous nature lies in their coming together with unusual severity.

St Thomas Aquinas uses similar categories, 'above nature',

'against nature', and 'besides nature', (*Summa Theol*, I, q 105, a 8; compare, *de Potentia* 6, 2, ad 3), but he is not sure into which category, for example, resurrection from the dead should go. In any event, this distinction is only relative to nature and not to the power of God.

Healing miracles form a convenient group for study from the scientific point of view because on their natural side they can be inspected with the tools of a fairly precise science; though Chapter V will indicate that the boundaries of this science are not nearly as precise as was once thought. But there is no intention here of supposing that 'healing miracles' are in a class apart from nature miracles. Such a distinction would be nonsense to any Biblical writer, and indicates an intolerably high-handed approach to the natural order.

It might be asked why Christians should be so concerned with miracles. Have we not got past that sort of thing in this modern scientific age? In a recent conversation a Christian psychiatrist dismissed them as 'a lot of ancient myths' which apparently had no relevance either to his religion or to his medicine.

However hostile the climate of opinion, Christians cannot back out in the matter of miracle. The theology of the Bible is concerned with material things. The doctrine of creation presupposes something very like a miracle in the beginning, and man occupies a special place in God's creation. If creation is one sphere of God's activity, history is another, and the Bible claims to be witness to the revelation of God in both. God's special activity in nature and history is focused to burning-point in miracle, and so this must be a cardinal point of concern for those who take God's self-revelation seriously.

This Judaeo-Christian concern for God's activity in this

world stands out the more sharply when contrasted with the disavowal of miracle by founders of other religions. Confucius refused to accept miracles. Buddha allowed only 'the miracles of the revelation of man's inner self'. For the Buddhist, doctrine *is* the miracle. Mohammed rejected miracles, claiming that the Koran only was miraculous. At the root of this rejection lies a devaluation of the material side of life which makes escape from matter to be of higher spiritual value than redemption of the whole world, matter included.

The main difficulties about miracle began to be experienced in Europe in the eighteenth century, but the attitude of extreme scepticism goes back at least as far as the Roman orator–philosopher Cicero (106–43 BC), who argued that since everything that happens has a cause, 'what was incapable of happening never happened, and what was capable of happening is not a miracle' (*De Divinatione*, 2, 28). But then Cicero, while a staunch supporter of the established religion, was philosophically an atheist. The argument is much more difficult than he would have us think. First we must examine the data.

2. Data and Assumptions of the Bible

A. OLD TESTAMENT

THE Old Testament never stops to argue the existence of God. He is its underlying presupposition, being the source of all life and all power. The fool can only say in his heart, 'There is no God' because God has given him the mind and breath to do so. The Israelites were not interested in science (in marked contrast with their contemporaries in Greece and the Greek Islands), and so they did not think in terms of a breach of natural order. God, being the creator of the world, can do what he likes; but he is faithful, that is to say reliable, and so the world is by and large a reliable place. Since God takes an intelligent interest in the running of his world, to put it at its lowest, he may be expected to adjust his acts to suit changing circumstances.

The contrast between the Hebrew and the Greek approach is illuminating. Both looked for a principle of coherence behind the changing face of things: the Greeks found it in orderliness and so called the world *kosmos*; the Hebrews found it in power, with God at the top of the power structure and the dead at the bottom, with gradations of more or less powerful spirits and people in between.

The Greeks set out to discover what a thing is, and then they would know how it behaves. For the Hebrews God is in control, and if he chooses to do mighty works these are 'natural' in that they accord with his reliability. No Hebrew

5

could have taken them as evidence for his existence. Israel was sure of God, and the world depended on him. The Greeks tried first to be sure about nature and thence discussed the place of God. The scope for the divine tended to be limited to what could not be ascribed to the orderliness of nature, a theory which laid itself open to all the difficulties of the 'God of the gaps'. In particular it is hard to use a divine 'intervention' which is a breach of natural orderliness as itself the basis of that orderliness. The Hebrews never doubted God's existence; they sought to interpret God's nature from his acts which were in history and concerned people—though they might well concern natural events as well.

The classic pattern of God's love in action was the Exodus from Egypt, an episode compounded of God's steadfast love for his people under oppression, his choice of them for future responsibility, his endowment of their leader, Moses, with special power for the task, his disfavour shown to their enemies by a series of plagues, even his hardening of a recalcitrant Pharaoh's heart, and finally his miraculous deliverance of his people by providing a dry passage for them across the 'Red Sea' and engulfing the pursuing Egyptian army. It is important to note that the writer of Exodus sees no contradiction between God's special personal activity here and the ordinary, or extraordinary, course of nature, for 'Moses stretched out his hand over the sea; and the Lord caused the sea to go back by a strong east wind all the night, and made the sea dry land . . .' (Exod 14.21).

The notion of nature as wholly self-governing was impossible for a Hebrew. They were not interested in an unbiased account of what happened. Their main interest in recording any happening lay in the bias which they thought it contained. The Greeks may have played with billiard balls; the Hebrews preferred bowls. It was the bias which made the game.

A year or two ago the name 'almoner' was removed from hospital vocabulary and 'medical social worker' substituted. We may regret the cacophony, but welcome the new insight which has recognised, after a century of scientific medicine, that, in the familiar words of John Donne, 'no man is an island unto himself'. If we had paid more attention to the Old Testament picture of man we would never have let ourselves be carried into the excessive individualism of nineteenth-century theory, which examined the organs of a sick man in detail but neglected his family and other relationships.

The word 'covenant' or 'testament' in the Bible expresses the deepest form of voluntary association between two people or parties. 'Then Jonathan and David made a covenant, because he loved him as his own soul' (I Sam 18.3). The characteristic unit of Israelite life is the family, and the nation is only a family writ large. It is a living organism in which the parts cohere, both giving and receiving strength and purpose. The nations often bear the names of their ancestors, as with Israel and Edom, named after Jacob (Israel) and Esau, and the family tree was not just names on paper but a lively organism stretching back into time towards, and in some sense still dependent upon, its founder. So God at the burning bush defines himself to Moses as 'Yahweh, the God of your fathers, the God of Abraham, of Isaac, and of Jacob' (Exod 3.15).

God's family extends outwards to embrace all nations and backwards to the patriarchs. It also extends upwards in the realm of spirit in relationship to God who gave them birth, gave them their name, and embraced them in his covenant.

Within the family unit the father plays a vital role. The privilege of the Hebrew father to beget and to bless is a direct reflexion of the inmost nature of God himself, 'the Father, from whom every fatherhood in heaven and on earth is named' (Eph 3.14 RV margin). The father is head of his family, and sustains and is sustained by the family. The obedient father brings blessings upon his family. In the disobedient family, it is the father who bears the responsibility and punishment. To be an isolated individual, cut off from one's father's house, was the worst fate that could befall an Israelite, but he was certainly no less an individual for being a member of a community. The Hebrew concept of the community was such 'that it did not, and does not, lend itself to extreme forms of individualism, communism, or even of hierarchy, but embraces all these in subtle harmony' (21, 30).

Much of this idea of community is carried through to the New Testament and underlies, for example, St Paul's maturest thought in Colossians and Ephesians. Christ as the New Adam, by sharing in full on the cross the isolation caused by Adam's sin, reverses the work of the Old Adam. Christ is not only the redeemer of Christians, nor the redeemer of men's moral and religious lives. By his sharing the fullness of man's life and death he draws all humanity with him to heaven, where he is the final cosmic fulfilment of the purposes of his Father's creation.

The Hebrew way of looking at the composition of an individual man is as unfamiliar to the Western mind as his social setting, and very far removed from the well-worn compartments of mind, body and soul. Indeed the most striking feature of Israelite thought is that man is a totality, a psycho-physical whole, a 'soul-substance'. This soul-substance is found in various parts of his body, as also in his shadow, his footprints, even his clothes. His personality is as extended as his family life.

The key-word in Hebrew psychology is *nephesh*, which defies translation. It probably comes from a root meaning neck or throat (see Is 5.14), and so is connected with breath, and comes to mean 'life', the common vital principle of man and beast. Life was located in the blood, and so at death it was either breathed out, or poured out. A great variety of emotional states are ascribed to *nephesh*, so that it ends up by being equivalent to 'self'. It passes on to mean 'a living person', and ends up occasionally as a 'dead one', i.e. a corpse. Such a term as *nephesh* would be the despair of a Greek philosopher.

As a man's *nephesh* (life or soul) was constantly in a state of ebb and flow, so also was his spirit, his vitality (*ruah*), which like the wind (which appears to be its root meaning) may range from gale force to whispering breeze. Again, *ruah* has two poles of meaning. On the physical side it can mean little more than breath. So with the Queen of Sheba on seeing Solomon's treasure, 'there was no longer any *ruah* in her' (I Kgs 10.5)—it took her breath away. On the psychical side it can denote almost any mood of feeling, disposition of heart, or frame of mind (as we say).

The more psychical powers are sometimes attributed to Yahweh. He is spirit and not flesh (Is 31.3); he is the author and sustainer of 'the spirits of all flesh' (Num 16.22), hovering over the cosmic waters at the creation of the world (Gen 1.2). God's spirit may fall upon a person and make him feel that he is in the hand of God, carried away in an ecstatic experience (Ezek 3.14); or again it may endow the ideal servant of Yahweh with the quiet wisdom necessary for God's ruling representative on earth (Is 11.2). In short, it is through spirit that a man's will is expressed for better or for worse; the ideal being that a man's spirit should be in harmony with the spirit of Yahweh (Ps 51.10–12).

That man is a psycho-physical organism is further illustrated by the way in which the Hebrews spoke of parts of the body as engaged in some form of personal behaviour. The head can receive blessing or responsibility for shed blood; the tongue can speak justice or slander; the eye is capable of pride or favour or hope, or their opposites; the arm is the main source of strength, for offence or defence; one's right hand is the principal pointer to one's feelings or intentions and the means for communicating these, be it blessing, cooking, offering, building, ruling, hitting, or killing.

One's internal parts are equally significant. Bones shrivel up with despondency or become soft with fear or distress, or are aflame with one's conflicting thoughts, or break up under the gnawing action of jealousy, and bone-marrow is felt to be enriched upon hearing good news. Blood is of vital significance because it contains the life-principle. So all blood is taboo for man and must be reserved for sacrifice to Yahweh. Even after death blood may retain its potency, as the blood of murdered Abel cried out against Cain.

The belly is the scene of profound emotional disturbances and also the repository of a person's basic motives. A man's loins, the source of his strength and procreative power, seem to collapse under strong agitation or apprehension. The bowels are stirred with feelings of love or despair, and the kidneys reveal similar extremes of emotional disturbance. The reins, indeed, conceal the real 'I'.

The most important, and the most-mentioned, organ, however is the heart (*lēbhabh*). The Israelites knew nothing of the circulation of the blood, but they were well aware of the heart's central importance, and it takes the place of the brain as the focal point of all psychical activity—what we should call 'mind' or 'intellect', the governing factor in one's behaviour. The Old Testament looks for 'purity' or 'integrity' of heart, and finds it in conformity with the will of Yahweh, for Yahweh looks not upon a man's outward appearance, but upon his heart. The crookedness of man's heart is due mainly to deceit or pride, and such a heart has either turned to fat or stone, and needs renewing.

Thus the Israelite saw a man not as a union of body and soul but as a psycho-physical organism, a unit of vital power, with vital extensions outside that unit. Death, however, breaks up the unity of the whole. It does not mean his complete extinction (even his name carried something of his personality), but death is a weak form of life. A dead person continues a shadowy existence in Sheol, but it is a 'land of darkness and deep shadow, the land of dusk-like gloom, of deep shadow and disorder' (Job 10.21–22), where a man is cut off from fellowship with Yahweh and so from the source of real life.

Even here the distinction is not clear-cut. Any weakness in life is a form of death, just as death itself is the weakest form of life. The distinction between 'living and partly living' is thoroughly Hebraic. Life for an Israelite meant a long, full, untroubled and prosperous life which included fruitfulness of body, flocks, soil, and commerce, together with national safety. Yahweh is the living God, the giver of life, and to enjoy good health and material prosperity is to walk with him in fullness of life.

It follows that the Israelite interpreted sickness in terms rather of Yahweh's disfavour than of organic disorder. The theory that piety brings prosperity and impiety disaster is worked out bluntly in Deuteronomy, with a good deal of squeezing of facts to fit the theory. The theory is somewhat modified by Jeremiah and Ezekiel, and meets its strongest opposition in the book of Job, where Job scorns the pious platitudes of his comforters, and at the end has his protest upheld by Yahweh. This drama gives no answer to the problem of unmerited suffering. Job is finally given a vision of the majesty of God in the created order of nature, and then realises that his question has lost its meaning.

In Job, as elsewhere in the Old Testament, illness is the work of Satan, though Satan is still one of God's faithful servants, loyally patrolling the earth. Similarly Saul's melancholia, which followed upon his disobedience and God's rejection of him, is ascribed to 'an evil spirit from God' (I Sam 16.15).

This approach to illness, that forgiveness was the prime need, must have militated against the work of the doctor, of whom we hear little in the Old Testament. King Asa suffered a severe disease in his feet, and receives the withering comment, 'yet in his disease he sought not to the Lord, but to the physicians' (2 Chron 16.12). The highest praise for the physician is in the Apocryphal book Ecclesiasticus (38.1–15), but even there the sick man is bidden 'pray unto the Lord and he shall heal thee. Put away wrong doing, and order thine hands aright. And cleanse thy heart from all manner of sin. . . . Then give place to the physician, for verily the Lord hath created him'.

The rigid causal connexion between sin and suffering was certainly still current in the time of Christ and equally certainly was repudiated by him. The victims of the Tower of Siloam disaster (Lk 13.1–5) were not worse offenders than the run of Jerusalem's inhabitants; and the man born blind (Jn 9.3) was not in this plight because of his own sins or those of his parents. In each case God is involved in the situation but not as punishing men for sins. Elsewhere Jesus points to some connexion between sin and disease—in the case of the paralysed man (Mk 2.3–12)—but this will receive fuller treatment later (see pp. 120f.).

Throughout the Old Testament all spirits, good and bad, are firmly under the control of Yahweh. But after the Exile Judaism radically altered its world view, suffering from a failure of nerve. The Jews had experienced a succession of foreign overlords. Prophecy had ceased. Miracles had ceased. What was God doing to allow his chosen people to be so ground down? Had he ceased to love them? Or was he not in final control? They could not give up faith in their election, but they did give up strict belief in Yahweh's sovereignty. So Satan and his fellow spirits 'fell' from being loyal servants of God to being evil demons setting up a rival kingdom of their own. The inter-testamental literature is full of accounts of the fall of angels—two in the Book of Enoch and another in the Book of Jubilees. The picture of a cosmos in revolt, a physical world corrupted and enslaved by God's enemy, is the theme of much apocalyptic literature.

The process may well have been helped by the thoroughgoing dualism of Persian religion with which the Exiles must have been in contact. Zoroastrianism presents a battle between two equal and opposite powers of good and evil. This kind of dualistic language is found in the New Testament, but it is never absolute—the kingdom in the last resort is always God's, and the final victory is his.

In general, apocalyptic literature was pessimistic about this world. The world was in the power of the Devil, doomed and without hope: the end would break in from outside in sheer catastrophe; but bodies would be resurrected and earth and heaven would be renewed. There is one remarkable exception to this picture, unique in the Bible, in the Apocryphal book *The Wisdom of Solomon*. This was probably written in Alexandria in the first century BC to encourage faithful Jews under persecution and to commend their religion by presenting the acts of their God in terms of the divine wisdom working itself out in history.

In particular the last chapter of *Wisdom* presents a theory of miracles in terms familiar to current late-Greek philosophy. It is that they are 'not a derangement but a re-arrangement of the harmony of the universe . . . and that these re-arrangements take place in accordance with, and to reveal, the moral principles on which the world is built'. Concerning the crossing of the Red Sea (19.6) the author comments, 'For the whole creation, each part in its several kind, was fashioned again anew, ministering to thy several commandments, that thy servants might be guarded free from hurt' (quotations from RV), and later (19.18) 'For as the notes of a psaltery vary the character of the rhythm, even so did the elements, changing their order one with another, continuing always the same, each in its several sound . . .' This reflects the interchange of what Greek philosophy regarded as the four basic elements, earth, air, fire and water (so also in 16.16–19).

Here is a bold attempt to combine the Hebrew picture of God who created the world out of nothing and controls it by his word, with the Greek theory that the world was shaped by God out of pre-existing matter and runs according to the unchangeable laws then provided. The word 'wisdom' appealed to the Greek sense of reason, but it was so highly personified that it is equivalent to God's word or hand. St Paul had no hesitation in taking it as one of his titles for Christ (I Cor 1.24). The emphasis of the book is not on the future, as it is in apocalyptic, but rather on the past and present: the final coming (Parousia) is not so much a future event as the ability to see things as they really are. In apocalyptic, miracles give pictures of the future; in *Wisdom*, they give meaning to the present. We shall see that in the New Testament both strains are to be found but by far the stronger is the present one.

The author of *Wisdom* is so keen to draw moral lessons from the miracles he recalls that he runs on to the shoals of allegory: we may not properly think of his transmutation of elements in terms of atomic physics. But he did make a valiant attempt to hold together a rational view of the uniformity of the world in the scientific terms of his day with the religious insight of God as its creator. To maintain both the immanence and the transcendence of God never has been an easy task.

B. NEW TESTAMENT

MIRACLES in the gospels can hardly be ignored, if only on account of their bulk. In St Mark's gospel 31 per cent of the whole, 209 out of 666 verses, is taken up with miracle stories: in his first ten chapters the proportion is as high as 47 per cent. St Mark without miracle is indeed Hamlet without the prince. The same is true, if not so mathematically, with St John's gospel. The first half (chapters 1–11) is well called 'the book of signs' where St John arranges his main themes around selected miracles; though it is hard to say where the narrative itself ends and the evangelist's comment begins. Such a modern distinction would not have worried St John.

We shall assume for the moment that the gospel narratives

are, broadly speaking, reliable historical documents; that
the miracle stories depend originally on eye-witnesses who
passed on their witness by word of mouth; that these
records came gradually to be crystallised in the young
Christian communities, not out of a desire for academic
history, but from pressing and practical demands of worship and teaching; that collections of sayings of the Lord
soon came to be written down; that the first gospel to be
published was that of St Mark about AD 65–70, being an
expansion of the earliest traditional preaching (*kērygma*);
that the gospels of St Matthew and St Luke followed in the
next twenty years, each based on St Mark, and each in-
corporating material from an early written collection mainly
of the sayings of the Lord (familiarly known as 'Q'); and
that the fourth gospel, bearing the name and authority of
the beloved disciple, completes and complements the series
with a profound interpretation of the person and work
of Jesus. A closer examination of the historical reliability of
the miracle stories in the gospels, especially in the light of
Form Criticism, is reserved until Chapter 6, pages 111–116.

Extra-biblical evidence is very slight—a reference to Jesus
who 'worked miracles, wonderful and mighty' in the
Slavonic translation of Josephus' *History of the Jewish War*,
but this is probably a medieval addition; and a Rabbinic
tradition in *Tractate Sanhedrin*, 43a, referring to a 'Yeshu of
Nazareth' who 'practised sorcery and beguiled and led
astray Israel' whom they hanged on the eve of the Passover.
The date of this is uncertain, but it may contain an independent Jewish tradition.

Within the New Testament but outside the gospels the
earliest witness to the Lord's miracles lies in the *kērygma*,
the pattern of the earliest apostolic preaching, which can be
deduced from a comparative study of the sermons in Acts.

This sketched in outline the birth of Jesus the Messiah, his ministry, his death, resurrection, ascension and spirit-giving, and ended with a challenge to the hearers to repent and join the new Messianic community by baptism. His ministry is described by St Peter (Acts 10.38 RV) in these terms, 'How that God anointed him with the Holy Ghost and with power: who went about doing good, and healing all that were oppressed of the devil; for God was with him'.

It was Christ's gift of the Spirit which enabled the church to continue works of healing by the same power which Christ had used. St Paul speaks of his own ministry as those things 'which Christ wrought through me, for the obedience of the Gentiles, by word and deed, in the power of signs and wonders, in the power of the Holy Ghost' (Rom 15.18f., RV). Similarly, the writer of the *Epistle to the Hebrews* speaks of the original eye-witnesses of the Lord having their words confirmed by 'signs and wonders, and with divers miracles, and gifts of the Holy Ghost' (Heb 2.3–4).

The strongest historical evidence, however, for the miracles of Jesus comes from his enemies. On many occasions Pharisees come into open conflict with him because of his works of power and the authority which he claims for doing them, but never do they cast any doubt on the fact that they were done. One charge at his trial concerned a miracle, the destruction and rebuilding of the temple, (Mk 14.58), and King Herod at his interrogation of Jesus hoped for a private display of miracle (Lk 23.8). It is hard to think that these charges would have been made if Jesus had been nothing but a travelling teacher.

Perhaps the most salutary lesson which has emerged from a century of Biblical scholarship is that we must guard against importing our own presuppositions into the reading of the gospels. We must first ask, and try to answer, the

question 'What did this mean to its writers and first readers?'
before we can ask the further question, 'What does this
mean to us?' Every one of the 'Lives' of Jesus ends up by
giving us as much insight into the mind of the author as
into the purposes of Christ.

That is why we have considered in some detail the Old
Testament background, because the New Testament is
written in a predominantly Hebraic idiom—although it is
written in Greek. To attempt to understand the healing
miracles in terms of nineteenth-century philanthropy is to
try measuring a patient's temperature with a slide-rule. In
fact, compassion for a sick person is never in the gospels
a primary motive for Jesus' healing. A reference to Jesus'
being moved with compassion occurs only three times in
St Mark, twice in the context of feeding miracles (6.34 and
8.2), and once of the healing of a leper (1.41); (but in the
last the reading of the Greek is uncertain, and the alternative *orgistheis* 'being angry' is probably preferable to
splanchnistheis as being the more difficult reading). St Luke,
strangely enough (for his is commonly thought to be the
humanitarian gospel), omits all St Mark's references to
compassion: St Matthew gives it most prominence (see
20.34; 14.14).

Nor may we look to the miracles for proof of Jesus'
divinity, although this has been the stock in trade of Christian
apologetic for many centuries. When accused by the
Pharisees of casting out demons by Beelzebub, prince of the
demons, Jesus is happy to acknowledge that God's healing
power is as much operative through their own exorcists as
it is through himself—'If I by Beelzebub cast out devils, by
whom do your sons cast them out?' (Mt 12.27). St Mark
records a complaint made by John, 'Master, we saw one
casting out devils in thy name: and we forbade him, because

he followed not us. But Jesus said, Forbid him not: for there is no man which shall do a mighty work in my name, and be able lightly to speak evil of me' (Mk 9.38–39). Jesus not only disowns the closed-shop mentality among his disciples, but makes a significantly close connexion between healing done in Jesus' name and an assessment of Jesus as a person.

Nor should we use miracles as an exercising-ground for the latest fashion in psychological theories, either for or against. 'They were all done by suggestion.' Some otherwise responsible writers go astray in this respect. When Alan Richardson writes, 'We stand entirely outside the New Testament edifice of faith and worship, if we assume that the miracles of Jesus are to be placed in the same category as the successes of modern psychotherapy, as merely illustrating the general truth of the supremacy of mind over matter or any other modern theory', he is more accurate about the New Testament than about psychotherapy (*41*, 137). But more of this in chapter 5.

The only proper categories through which the New Testament miracles can be approached and assessed are those of the Old Testament. The very words for 'miracle' are Old Testament words. 'Miracle' is an unfortunate translation, as it puts primary emphasis on the wonder caused. In the Synoptic (that is, the first three) gospels the most important word is *dynamis* ([work of] power), which fits naturally the Hebrew dynamic conception of God who can (Greek, *dynatai*) do all things. The other main word is *sēmeion* (sign) corresponding to the Hebrew '*ôth*. In the Synoptic gospels *sēmeion* usually has a bad meaning— of a sign asked for as a proof; but in St John it reverts to the Old Testament usage of a sign pointing beyond itself to God's wonders. St John is also fond of the word *ergon* meaning 'deed' or 'work', with Hebraic emphasis on activity and concreteness. The ordinary word for a 'wonder' (Greek *teras*) is not found in the Synoptics. The phrase 'signs and wonders' is occasionally used reputably (e.g. Acts 2.22) *sēmeia kai terata*, but this is an echo of the Old Testament *'ôthôth w^emôph^ethîm*. Three other words occur once each, *thaumasia* (Mt 21.15); *paradoxa* (Lk 5.26); *aretai* (I Pet 2.9).

A standing warning is spoken to those who neglect Old Testament antecedents in the words addressed to the two disciples by the risen Lord on the road to Emmaus, 'Behoved it not the Christ to suffer these things, and to enter into his glory?' (Lk 24.26), as also in those to the Sadducees, 'Is it not for this cause that ye err, that ye know not the Scriptures, nor the power (*dynamis*) of God?' (Mk 12.24).

'But if I by the finger of God cast out devils, then is the kingdom of God come upon you' (Lk 11.20). In this decisive claim there are three important items. First, Jesus himself acts with the power of God (finger of God is a Hebraism, strangely preserved by the Gentile St Luke, in contrast to St Matthew who has 'spirit of God'). Second, the casting out of devils, which is not unique to Jesus, marks the overthrow of cosmic forces of evil. Third, this crisis marks the beginning of the establishment of God's kingdom.

The theme of the kingdom of God is the *leit-motif* of the Synoptic gospels (transposed in St John into 'eternal life'). It figures in the opening proclamation of the good news by Jesus according to St Mark, 'The time is fulfilled, and the kingdom of God is at hand: repent ye, and believe in the gospel' (Mk 1.15). It is the theme of the majority of the Lord's parables. It is the charge on which he is finally condemned (Mk 15.2) and which is nailed above him on the cross (Mk 15.26). It lies at the heart of the Lord's prayer, and is there defined in typical Hebrew parallelism—'thy kingdom come; thy will be done'. God's kingdom is not a place but is his reign recognised and accepted. It is so in heaven, and it can be so on earth.

The gospel is the good news that the long period of waiting is over. 'Today hath this scripture been fulfilled in your ears' (Lk 4.21, RV). The scripture which Jesus chooses in the Nazareth synagogue concerns the anointed (Greek *christos*) servant of Yahweh who is commissioned

> '. . . to preach good tidings to the poor:
> He hath sent me to proclaim release to the captives,
> And recovering of sight to the blind,
> To set at liberty them that are bruised,
> To proclaim the acceptable year of the Lord.'
> (Lk 4.18f., RV, quoted from Is 61.1–2)

In much the same terms Jesus answers John the Baptist's question whether he is the expected Messiah: 'Go your way and tell John the things which ye do hear and see: the blind receive their sight, and the lame walk, the lepers are cleansed, and the deaf hear, and the dead are raised up, and the poor have good tidings preached to them' (Mt 11.4–5. RV). This healing mission may have been meant metaphorically by Isaiah; for Jesus it is actual and visible. Again, Jesus tells the disciples that they are seeing and hearing the things which many prophets and righteous men desired to see and hear but could not (Mt 13.17).

Jesus, in his person, and by his acts, proclaimed the coming of the kingdom. The point was not lost on his enemies and St Mark portrays their opposition very early in his gospel (Mk 2.1–12). Jesus is confronted by a paralysed man brought to him by four friends. Jesus pronounces his

sins forgiven. The scribes understandably call this blasphemy for such authority belongs only to God. Jesus
reinforces his claim by healing the paralysed man. The
crowd of bystanders take the point and glorify God who
(St Matthew adds) had given such power unto men (Mt.
9.8).

The Pharisees cannot—or do not—deny his miracles.
They can only accuse him of using Satan's power in doing
them (see Mt 12.24f. Lk 11.15f.). Jesus answers that their
very charge implies that Satan's power is overthrown, his
kingdom split, his castle captured. Later, after the return of
the seventy from their mission, his mysterious statement, 'I
beheld Satan fallen as lightning from heaven' (Lk 10.18)
again seems to proclaim a decisive defeat for the kingdom of
evil and victory for the kingdom of God.

Jesus' miracles, then, can never be separated from his
proclamation of the kingdom. By his miracles he proclaims,
portrays, and initiates the kingdom of God.

The ability by which men respond to this proclamation
and accept or enter the kingdom is faith. This ability may
be divine in origin, but it requires man's response to make it
effective. To enter the kingdom is to be saved, and the
phrase 'thy faith hath saved thee' is characteristic of the
miracle stories. The word 'save' (Greek *sōzein*) with its noun
'salvation' (Greek *sōtēria*) has a rich background of
meaning, and within the New Testament a wide variety. It is
used 102 times in the New Testament, 13 times in a medical
context and 73 in a theological context. There 'salvation' is
from the bondage of sin, sickness, meaninglessness, death
and judgment. It is also salvation into freedom, into health,
and into eternal life here and now. It is often eschatological,
that is, connected with the Day of the Lord.

Restoration to health was not the primary aspect of

salvation, though it was often an important secondary one. (The root meaning of the Hebrew word for 'salvation' is 'having room to develop'.) It is possible to receive miraculous healing and not be made whole. The ten lepers were cleansed of their leprosy; but only one, the Samaritan, who fell on his face at Jesus' feet and gave glory to God, was made whole by his faith (Lk 17.11–19, RV). It is equally possible to receive salvation from sin and alienation without physical sickness being present. Zacchaeus received salvation when he accepted Jesus into his house and accepted the fact that he was accepted by Jesus: no doubt the fit of generosity which accompanied his conversion was also beneficial to his health (Lk 19.1–10).

Faith was necessary for healing not because a cure was physically impossible without it, but because it would have been spiritually meaningless. When Jesus returned to Nazareth (Mk 6.1–6) and was flatly rejected by his own people, naturally 'he could there do no mighty work, save that he laid his hands upon a few sick folk, and healed them'. The notion that faith is 'a kind of psychological atmosphere . . . where the presence of the crowd, given that atmosphere, would increase suggestibility' is, *pace* Dr Weatherhead, an anachronism.

The predominant modern interest in healing miracles is in a private transaction between two people, healer and healed, with a possible extension to friends or relatives of the sick person. This is reflected in the normal pattern of the Church's ministry to the sick, as for example, the priest's bringing Holy Communion to a sick person at home with perhaps one or two friends present. The individualism underlying this is as alien to the New Testament conception of miracles as it is to the Old Testament conception of man.

The coming of the kingdom, that is to say the coming of

Jesus, presents the nation with a crisis, that is (in the literal translation of the Greek *krisis*) judgment. The preaching of the gospel, or better, the proclaiming of the good news, and the healing of the sick are not two separate items in the programme; they are different aspects of the same thing: the preaching, especially in the parables of the kingdom, explains its nature and the response to which it challenges its hearers, that is, repentance. The healing of people *is* the kingdom come with saving and power. It is worth remembering that the Hebrew word *dābhār* means both 'word' and 'deed'. This combination of healing and preaching which is the heart of Jesus' ministry is continued in the mission of the disciples. Jesus' charge to them as they go out is recorded four times in the Synoptic gospels (Mk 6.7–13; Mt 9.35–10.23; Lk 9.1–6; and Lk 10.1–20), and in each account preaching and healing are conjoined. St Mark sums up the mission, 'And they went out, and preached that men should repent. And they cast out many devils, and anointed with oil many that were sick, and healed them'. St Matthew says, 'And as ye go, preach, saying, The kingdom of heaven is at hand. Heal the sick, raise the dead, cleanse the lepers, cast out devils: freely ye received, freely give'. St Luke, in the charge to the seventy, records, 'Heal the sick . . . and say unto them, The kingdom of God is come nigh unto you'.

The authority which Jesus has claimed for his own healing work, the power of God, the action of the Holy Spirit, he here delegates to his apostles. They are to act as his ambassadors, and miracles are to be their credentials as they were his. Further, the reception accorded to them is in fact reception accorded to him, and is thus reception accorded (or refused) to God, the author of all mission. St Luke ends the Lord's charge to the seventy, 'He that heareth you heareth me; and he that rejecteth you rejecteth

me; and he that rejecteth me rejecteth him that sent me'
(Lk 10.16). The same note is struck in St Matthew 10.40 and
St John 13.20, that to receive the apostles is to receive Jesus
and so to receive God. Miracles are signs of judgment as
well as signs of love.

Here we must break away from a Western individualistic
way of thinking and try to understand the healing miracles
in their corporate and representative setting.

First, Jesus is himself Representative Man. By his incarnation he identified himself with human flesh, human
personality; by his baptism he identified himself with
human sinfulness, though himself without sin (Mt 3.13–
17); by his title Son of Man he acknowledged full humanity,
rejected the political image of a Davidic Messiah and
accepted instead that of a Suffering Servant; and by his death
he fulfilled the vocation of Israel. The idea of Christ as
Representative Man is familiar in Christian thinking about
the Atonement, and evidence for it can be gathered from
almost every writer in the New Testament, but very little
thought has been given to the representative aspect of his
ministry. The most striking passage where he identifies
himself with every man in need is the parable of the sheep
and goats. Any visit paid to a sick person is a visit paid
to Christ, 'Inasmuch as ye did it unto one of these my
brethren, even these least, ye did it unto me' (Mt 25.40 RV).
The taunt 'Physician, heal thyself' (Lk 4.23), like the taunt
'Come down from the cross' (Mk 15.30), shows how Jesus
identified himself with sick and sinful humanity.

Further, if Jesus the healer was himself representative of
the community, the sick whom he healed were also its
representatives. Jesus carefully selects those whom he healed;
he certainly could not heal all who were sick, or he would
have no time for the other parts of his work, or for rest.

Even so untheological a writer as St Mark sees a kind of progression in the early works of healing: the first healing is in the synagogue, the heart of the worshipping community (1.21); then in Peter's home (1.30); on to the Jewish city (1.33); to the Jewish outcast (1.40); and later, with the Syro-Phœnician woman's daughter (7.29) to the Gentile world. Blind Bartimaeus (Mk 10.46–52) who is given his sight, is contrasted with the blind disciples, who immediately before were quarrelling about precedence, and with the blind crowd who immediately after hail Jesus as Messiah but with no understanding of the meaning of that title. St John works out this theme with magnificent artistry in chapter 9 where the man born blind is shown to be the true representative of the community and receives his sight, whereas the Pharisees, who imagine themselves to be the true representatives of Israel, although they can see, are declared blind and sinful.

The significance of a healing miracle is not restricted to the one who heals and the one who is healed. Those who witness it are also important representatives of the community. 'Because of the multitude which standeth around I said it, that they may believe that thou didst send me.' So St John records Jesus' words after the raising of Lazarus (Jn 11.42), and even if they are not *ipsissima verba* of the Lord, they are a fair summary of the situation. Of course, Jesus refused to do a miracle simply to impress people, but similarly he did not heal people just to make them better. He healed them so that they and those who witnessed the healing, should by it be moved to respond to the challenge of the kingdom which they had personally experienced. Even Lazarus had to die again. But 'he that believeth on me, though he die, yet shall he live: and whosoever liveth and believeth on me shall never die' (Jn 11.25–26 RV).

One of the more baffling aspects of the healing stories of the gospels is their frequent description in terms of demon-possession and demon-expulsion (exorcism). A glance is needed at the origin of these unfamiliar concepts.

Belief in demons, we have already said (p. 13f), became widespread in Israel in the post-exilic period under Babylonian influence, and represented a serious threat to the sovereignty of Yahweh, especially as possession was a matter of chance and not the result of wrongdoing. By the third century AD Judaism was swamped with demons. Rabbi Johanan (died 279) knew of three hundred varieties of demon, and it was said that everyone had a thousand to his left and a hundred thousand to his right.

The origin of demons was ascribed to the fall of angels. The Book of Enoch declares that in the days of Jared two hundred sons of heaven came down to Mount Hermon, inflamed by desire for the fair daughters of earth (see Gen 6.1f.). Such a theory was accepted without question by such a variety of theologians as Origen, St Thomas Aquinas and Calvin. These fallen angels taught the women charms and spells, and instructed them in the cutting of roots and the quest for medicinal herbs. A clear link is here made between demons and witchcraft. Their homes were places of terror, especially the desert, but also water, wind, graves and ruins. The task of demons was to lead men astray in every respect, and for Rabbis of the post-Christian era each disease was caused by a particular demon. As supernatural creatures they also possessed supernatural knowledge.

Defence against demons lay in various magic rites, recipes, charms, and incantations. The sprinkling of blood at passover (Exod 12.22) is the relic of a rite to ward off a destroying spirit, dating from a time before the transformation of the feast by Moses. Isaiah 3.20 mentions amulets as an item of jewellery; Egypt has produced a mass of papyri with magical formulae used by Jews of the late post-Exilic period; the Book of Tobit (chapters 6 and 7) gives an angelic recipe of the liver and heart of a fish to be burned in order to drive away a demon of death.

Against such a background Jesus did his healing miracles, and it is hardly surprising that they are couched in terms familiar to his day. This is not just an accommodation to the needs of his hearers, but the inevitable consequence of the incarnation accepted to its depths. Jesus addressed demons as if they were in possession of a man, ordering them to come out and free the victim: 'Hold thy peace and come out of him' to the madman in the Capernaum synagogue (Mk 1.25; see also Mk 5.8; Mk 9.25; Mt 8.32; Lk 4.35). And they did.

What is more perplexing is the fact that demons, using their supernatural knowledge, recognise Jesus where men have failed to do so. 'I know thee who thou art, the Holy One of God' (Mk 1.24); 'Thou art the Son of God' (Mk 3.11); 'Jesus, thou Son of the Most High God' (Mk 5.7). Wrede, the radical German scholar, at the turn of the century dismissed this as a literary device to let readers of the gospel into the secret of Jesus' identity from the outset. Other scholars suggest clairvoyance on the lines of the Delphic oracle. Others see a heightened awareness of a person in a trance. Yet another, Bauernfeind, ingeniously suggests that the madman is using stock defensive magic words to repel what he fears to be an attack by yet another exorcist: this would be his strongest weapon, and would be suitable for one suffering from paranoia. We have not really enough evidence to come to a clear decision.

Do demons really exist? Jaspers, the existentialist philosopher, says, 'There are no such things as demons'. He describes the exorcisms of Jesus as 'the historical form of an existentially experienced reality'. William Temple wrote of Satan, 'Personally I believe he exists and that a large share of that responsibility (for human evil) belongs to him and to subordinate evil spirits'. Perhaps asking the question (Do demons exist?) is, logically speaking, like asking the question 'Do nervous breakdowns exist?' Thousands of people have had nervous breakdowns and will describe the medical treatment they have had for them. Yet any psychiatrist will fight shy of using this expression. He would describe the patient as suffering from a neurosis, or perhaps a psychosis, and could further sub-divide this under various heads; other authorities are now saying that the word 'neurosis' is misleading because it locates the trouble in the nerves, and are advocating the word 'sociosis', which would locate the trouble in personal relationships, instead. Someone has written a book denying that there is such a thing as 'mental illness' at all!

Which all goes to show how hard it is to talk in a clear and common language about the deep things of the personality. What is obvious today is that we have no adequate map of the human person, and much confusion is caused by cross-talk. (Compare p. 70 on the question 'Do miracles happen?')

A more important question to ask is, What conviction were the evangelists concerned to express when they spent so much time recording Jesus' healing of demon-possessed people? It was a coherent part of the gospel; the good news that the decisive time had come; that a decisive conflict was in progress between the powers of the kingdom and the powers of evil; and the powers of evil were being routed. The main contention of the New Testament, especially in the Pauline epistles, with regard to demons is not that they do not exist or that they are unreal, but that the power of Christ, which is the power of God's kingdom, has conquered them: (see for example Eph 1.20–23 or Col 1.12–13 RV, 'giving thanks unto the Father . . . who delivered us out of the power of darkness, and translated us into the kingdom of the Son of his love'.)

The number of exorcisms which Jesus did on the Sabbath is significant. This was not just to bait the Pharisees, a deliberate seeking for trouble; it was the renewal of God's creation, a new bringing of order out of chaos. 'Ought not this woman, being a daughter of Abraham, whom Satan hath bound, lo, these eighteen years, to have been loosed from this bond on the day of the sabbath?' (Lk 13.16). Jesus maintains that God's creative activity was visible in a new and personal way in his works: 'But Jesus answered them, My Father worketh even until now, and I work. For this cause therefore the Jews sought the more to kill him, because he not only brake the sabbath, but also called God his own Father, making himself equal with God.' (Jn 5.17–18 RV). The Greek word with which Jesus rebukes the demon in the possessed man in the Capernaum synagogue 'Hold thy peace' (Mk 1.25; Greek, *phimōthēti*) is the same as that addressed to the storm on the lake 'Peace, be still' (Mk 4.39; Greek, *pephismo*). Both were addressed to a world gone berserk; both brought order out of chaos, as the divine word brought order out of chaos on the first day of creation.

It may be that today we should look for demonic powers at work in fields wider than individual sickness. Tillich speaks of demonic powers in national political life, and Jung said he was compelled to believe in demonic possession in the light of Nazi German atrocities. If all human personal illness were healed (and this is a scientific possibility), social sickness would remain. Demons would still need to be exorcised.

Miracles, if they are to be a part of the self-revelation of God, must be consistent with all that is known from other sources about him. In particular, if Jesus Christ is the focal point of God's self-revelation, then his miracles must be consistent not only with the rest of his life and teaching, but also with the deepest insights of the Old Testament into the personal being of God. Is this so?

Miracles are the credentials of an ambassador which point beyond the bearer to the power whom he represents. Therefore miracles can never be self-seeking. At his temptation in the wildnerness Jesus became vividly aware of the treasonable possibilities of miracle—to satisfy his own hunger for food, or popularity, or power (Mt 4.1–11).

> The last temptation is the greatest treason:
> To do the right deed for the wrong reason.

'Beware of false prophets, which come to you in sheep's clothing, but inwardly are ravening wolves. . . . Many will say to me in that day, Lord, Lord, did we not prophesy by thy name, and by thy name cast out devils, and by thy name do many mighty works? And then will I profess unto them, I never knew you: depart from me, ye that work iniquity' (Mt 7.15–23). It is apparent from warnings in the Epistles that some early Christians supposed that godliness was a way of gain (see 1 Tim 6.5 and 2 Pet 2.3). The contrast with such heathen wonder-workers as Apollonius of Tyana, whose main concern was his remuneration, stands out sharply. The disciples were to give freely, for freely had they received (Mt 10.8).

The miracles that Jesus did *not* do are as impressive as

those that he did. Most notable was his refusal to do the final miracle of all, to save himself and come down from the cross. Such a miracle was a logical impossibility—as the priests who stood by mockingly observed, 'He saved others; himself he cannot save'.

Monden refers to moving passages from St Gregory of Nazianzus (a theme developed by many of the Fathers of the Church) describing how he who fed thousands with a few loaves fasted and knew hunger; he who promised to remove all weariness fell asleep in Peter's boat; he who had often restored speech to the dumb allowed himself to be led silent as a lamb to the slaughter; he who had put the demons to flight with a word handed himself over without protest to the powers of darkness; he who had healed the man born blind with his spittle allowed his eyes to be covered and spat upon; the healer of lepers became, according to the words of Isaiah, a leper, as one from whom men hide their face; his face which shone like the sun on Mount Tabor was marred, despised and rejected; the Master who changed water into wine accepted vinegar to quench his thirst. The Lord who raised Lazarus from the dead and restored her son to the widow of Nain went solitary into death, and left his mother alone to bear the burden of her grief.

The reticence of the miracle-narratives in the gospels stands out most clearly by contrasting them with the flowery products of later pious imagination. Christians felt that there were important gaps in the official gospels, particularly in the childhood of Christ, which needed filling, and soon plenty of miracles were found to fill them. The unofficial (or apocryphal) gospel of Thomas, for instance, tells how Jesus as a boy was being taught the alphabet, but his master was annoyed at the brilliance he showed and struck him on the head. Whereupon Jesus cursed him, and the master fell down and died. Again, when Jesus was six years old his mother sent him to draw water. But he broke his pitcher at the well. He took the cloak that he was wearing and filled that with water, and so brought it back to his mother. Or again, Joseph found that one of his planks of wood was too short, so Jesus tells him to hold one end while he holds the other, and so proceeds to pull it out to the required length (*13*, 63–64). The fictitious quality of these stories shouts aloud.

There is a notable reserve surrounding the miracles of Jesus. There is none of the strident technique of the advertiser about them. An advertiser is concerned only to sell his wares; these need in no way be connected with his own integrity as a person. The miracle-worker, however, must be a sign in himself as much as in his works; his own sanctity must be no different from that of his miracles, for both of them must point beyond themselves to God. So when the seventy return from their mission, thrilled with their victory over demons, Jesus cools their enthusiasm: 'In this rejoice not, that the spirits are subject unto you; but rather rejoice, because your names are written in heaven' (Lk 10.20). Their personal worthiness was not a matter of natural character or intellect, but was a God-given endowment. The failure of the disciples to heal the epileptic boy is attributed to their lack of prayer (Mk 9.28f.).

This reticence stands out again in contrast with the parade accompanying the wonder-workings of pagans like Apollonius of Tyana. There are no pompous processions or tricks; no hangers-on, no mediums; no hypnosis or suggestion; no complicated ceremonial; no Dionysiac ecstasy; no use of potions or drugs. Jesus avoids crowds and enthusiasm (see Jn 6.14f., of a crowd which wished to take him by force and make him a king; Mt 8.16–18; Mt 14.23;

Lk 5.15–16, etc.). Frequently he bids those whom he healed
to tell no one (see Mk 1.44–45; Mk 3.12; Mk 5.43; Mk 7.36;
Mk 8.26, etc.) because he was as well aware of the spiritual
danger of a magician Messiah as of the political danger of a
rebel Messiah. He rebukes the crowd (Jn 6.25f.) following
him because they saw the miracle of the loaves but failed to
see its meaning more deeply than in terms of bread and
hunger. Frequently he takes a sick person aside to heal him
(e.g. Mk 8.23, the blind man at Bethsaida); there is no
raising of voice, just two or three words of a peremptory
command, a simple gesture—and it is done. Monden sums
up these characteristics of Jesus' power as stemming from 'a
royal serenity, an almost careless majesty' (*33*, 110).

The uselessness of miracles for display purposes has been
illustrated pointedly and with great humour by Bruce
Marshall in his novel, *Father Malachy's Miracle* (*27*). A
zealous young priest in Edinburgh, Father Malachy
Murdoch, o.s.b., partly out of spite towards his sceptical
Episcopalian neighbour, and partly out of conviction that
the English-speaking peoples stand in need of supernatural
fireworks to bring them back to God, prays for a shattering
miracle. He asks that, on the Feast of the Translation of the
Holy House of Loretto, at 11.30 p.m., a nearby semi-un-
righteous dancing hall called *The Garden of Eden* shall be
removed to the Bass Rock in the Firth of Forth. It takes off
at the appointed moment, and at thirteen minutes to twelve
lands on the Rock, complete with its staff and patrons.

The police are in consternation, but they can find no law
against miracles. The miracle is widely discounted as the
product of auto-suggestion or mass hypnotism. An Anglican
dean laments miracles as being as much bad form as they are
bad science, and is glad that no Anglican clergyman would
have been allowed to perform one. Father Malachy gets into

trouble for not asking permission of his bishop, who maintains a guarded position. The bishop's brother had been there, in company with a dancing lady, but refused to believe that it had happened. The verdict of a cardinal is that if ecclesiastics were to make a habit of removing cabarets every time they exceeded the theological definition of chastity, the air would be filled with flying cabarets. 'We have enough to do to get people to swallow the necessary miracles without trying to pour down a few extra ones.'

Father Malachy is offered the serial rights of his miracle for cinema and press, and *The Garden of Eden*, turned into a luxury casino, becomes a brilliant, world-wide attraction. Father Malachy is persuaded by his rector that the only solution is to ask for its removal back again, and with a prayer that God would forgive the pride of a priest who had sought to effect in a day what his Saviour had failed to do in two thousand years, the hall is returned to its place. 'Perhaps', reflects the humbled priest, 'he allowed me to do it in order to show me that his ordinary means were best after all. . . . It is certainly a miracle that *The Garden of Eden* should be on the Bass Rock; but it is equally another miracle that the majority of people should refuse to believe that it is a miracle'.

In harmony with the whole of Christ's redemptive work, his miracles are exclusively of healing and re-creation, and never of maiming or destruction, at least as far as people are concerned. On the sub-human level there are recorded the destruction of the Gadarene swine (Mk 5.13) and the withering of the fig-tree (Mk 11.20), but the first may be understood as a popular interpretation added to the original healing story, and the second may be a parable transformed into a miracle.

Every miracle is set in a context of faith, and faith means

an awareness that in the event a personal and demanding claim was being made on behalf of the kingdom of God. If faith was wholly absent miracles could not be done (Mk 6.5), not because it was a physical impossibility, but because it was a logical impossibility; in such a context they would have been irrelevant. On such occasions there were many sick people whom Jesus could not (Mk 6.5) and did not (Mt 13.58) heal. There were others, too. Sometimes Jesus withdrew from pressing crowds because their demands were impeding the proclamation of the good news (Mk 1.38). So far as we can tell he saw his ministry as directed entirely to Jewish people, and the occasional healing of a Gentile is recorded as being very much an exception (as the Syro-Phœnician woman, Mk 7.24–30). The same limitation is applied to the mission of the disciples (Mt 10.5). Similarly Jesus refuses to 'lay on' a miracle to impress the Pharisees (Mt 12.38 f.) or Herod (Lk 23.8–9) or, in the greatest refusal of all, the chief priests (Mk 15.27–32).

'Faith' by no means implies, in the gospels, a conviction on the part of the sufferer that Jesus can heal him. In this respect it is very different from some modern kinds of 'faith-healing'. Sometimes the faith is more evidently possessed by friends or relatives of the sick person, as the four friends who brought the paralysed man to Capernaum (Mk 2.1–12), or the father of the epileptic boy (Mk 9.24). On every occasion Jesus seems to be confident that conditions are such that the miracle *may* be interpreted by those present as a sign of the presence and the power of the kingdom of God. There was always the risk that it might not be. Ten lepers were healed and went away; only one returned to Jesus to give thanks to God, and only one was saved (Lk 17.11–19).

Miracles, then, so far from being an optional extra to the

gospel, are an integral part of it. They are indeed spotlights which concentrate and focus the healing power of God, the complement to his message of salvation. 'We may demand of the miracles', with St Augustine, 'what they have to say to us of Christ; for they have, if they are rightly understood, a language of their own. For, because Christ himself is the Word of God, every action of that Word is equally a word spoken to us' (St Augustine, *In Johannem*, tract. 24,6).

3. The Place of Miracles in Christian Thought: A Historical Sketch

To MOVE into the sphere of popular Christian apologetic literature (that is, writings designed to defend the Christian cause) of the second and third centuries is like entering a world of science-fiction. It belongs to a world of fantasy, and lays no claim to real historical worth. Miracles are adduced to vindicate a martyr or provide divine proof of the truth of an apostle's preaching. According to the Acts of John (39f.) this apostle, preaching at Ephesus, challenges his audience to a trial of strength between Artemis and the Christian God, very much in the style of Elijah on Mount Carmel. St John and his cause are splendidly vindicated when the altar and statue of Artemis are overthrown and the temple roof finally collapses on her priest.

Since the ancient world was full of miracles wrought by gods and heroes, Christian apologists had to maintain the superiority of Christian ones. The defence by the serious apologists followed three lines—an appeal to the works of Christ; reference to the recorded miracles of the apostles; and claims for contemporary miracles. Athanasius in his *De Incarnatione* shows that Christ's miracles proclaim him Lord of Nature, greater than any man, master of demons, and by his resurrection, mightier than any hero. Upon these arguments two attacks were made: that the miracle stories were fictitious; or that the miracles were works of sorcery.

The first was answered by claiming contemporary witness for healings recorded in the gospels. Quadratus, the earliest apologist, writing about AD 124, is quoted by Eusebius the historian of the Church (iv, 3, 2) as saying, 'those who were healed or were raised from the dead were not only seen when they were being healed and raised from the dead, but they remained present not only during the life but also after the death of the Saviour, and indeed for a considerable time, so that some have come down even to our days'. (Though he does not show any close knowledge of such survivors.)

This argument ceased to exist after the next generation, and later apologists support the truth of miracles by connecting them with the moral excellence of the disciples, who were prepared to give their lives in defence of that truth, and who had spread the gospel from Persia to Britain. The argument that the miracles were in fact the work of demons was harder to rebut. In dealing with it Origen in the middle of the third century tends to spiritualise the miracle-stories almost out of existence, taking the healing of the blind and deaf to refer to all those who are having their eyes opened to the truth and their ears ready for the gospel (*Contra Celsum*, 2.48). In answer to the charge of sorcery, Origen points to the moral quality of the miracle. The proof of Jesus' works as divine is the creation of the Christian life, as the proof of the Resurrection is the life of the Christian church.

The appeal to miracles as a defence of the gospel's truth thus ends up as an appeal to the gospel as a defence of the miracles' truth—which is not surprising in view of our contention that miracle and gospel are not to be separated.

On the whole the early apologists tend to look back on miracles as things of the past—with one important exception: the matter of exorcism. The contemporary pagan world was densely populated with demons, and when these were cast out by Christians, or forced to declare their names, this was proof of the superiority of Christ to the pagan gods. Such exorcism was not always connected with miraculous acts of healing, but was generally part of the constant warfare with heathenism. It was to assume demonic proportions itself in later centuries.

For simpler souls the text 'with God all things are possible' may be a sufficient basis for understanding miracles, but as soon as miracles are used to justify the gospel, or the gospel is used to justify miracles, then large and difficult questions have to be asked.

Can God do everything? The stoics would tend to say that he can, that divine providence can mould matter in any shape needed. But the main line of platonic thought would deny it. Pliny states that God cannot die, give mortals immortality, recall the dead, change the past, or make twice ten not equal to twenty (*Natural History*, 2.27). Here we are confronted with the problem of the consistency of nature which is to be a central theme over the next eighteen centuries. Origen agrees with his opponent Celsus that God cannot go against nature, but what is 'against nature'? The early Christian thinkers did not forget that the primary Christian doctrine is of God as creator, and Tertullian (soon after AD 200) had to oppose Marcion for claiming that Christ's miracles showed him to be superior to, and in conflict with, the Creator-God of the Old Testament. So the miracles of Christ tended to be minimised.

In contrast, Gregory of Nyssa (towards the end of the fourth century) gives full value to the miracles of Christ, but like Origen, chooses to describe them as 'greater than nature'. Hilary of Poitiers (at about the same date) goes further, describing Christ as having a heavenly body, whose proper nature it is to walk on water (*de Trinitate*, 10.23). Here indeed lies the agonising difficulty of maintaining both the humanity and the divinity of Christ. Either the miracles prove too much, so that Christ ceases to be wholly human, or else they prove too little, in which case they cease to be miracles. But at least the early Fathers clung to the basic Christian assertions that the miracles are special signs of God the Creator whose unique acts in Christ are neverthe-less consistent with the total ordering of his creation.

Up to the time of St Augustine there had not been much close analysis of the subject of miracle. The climate of thought was mainly platonic and so concerned not so much with cause and effect as with the correspondence of things with their ideal model, from which followed an emphasis on their symbolic value. St Augustine, writing soon after AD 400 is the first to draw up a systematic doctrine of miracle, and its effect was to last until the end of the twelfth century. He puts so much emphasis on the sign-value of miracle that he almost neglects its transcendence. He sees divine inter-vention not so much as an act of God's creative power as an awakening of seeds already planted in things by the hand of Providence. In expounding the feeding of the five thousand he comments:

The miracles worked by our Lord are divine acts which rouse the human mind towards discerning God in things visible. God is not a substance visible to the eyes, and familiarity has bred such contempt for his miracles by which he rules the whole world and looks after the entire creation that scarcely anyone deigns to notice the wonderful and amazing works of God in a single grain of wheat. So, faithful to his mercy, he has reserved to himself certain things which he should do, in his own time, going beyond the usual course and order of nature, so that people to whom everyday things had become cheap might be amazed not by greater but by more unusual things. For the governing of the whole world is a greater miracle than the satisfying of five thousand with five loaves: yet nobody wonders at the former. They wonder at the latter not because it is greater but because it is unusual. For who is it who now feeds the whole world if it is not he who produces crops from a few grains? He acted therefore as God acts. From the source by which he multiplies crops from a few grains, from that same source he multiplied five loaves in his own hands (*In Johannis Evangelium*, 24.1).

Here is a clinging to the doctrine of creation with a vengeance!

How can anything be against nature that happens by the will of God, since the will of so great a maker is the nature of every made thing? A miracle, therefore, does not happen against nature, but against nature as it is known (*de Civitate Dei*, 21.8, 2).

St. Thomas Aquinas, however, sets a new pattern which was to be standard for the medieval Schoolmen. By his time the theological climate had profoundly changed. The platonism of the Fathers had yielded before the rediscovery in Western Europe of the works of Aristotle. Theology ceases to be reflexion within the faith, nourished with piety, and begins to seek the status of a science, based on reason, and thinking in terms of cause and effect. The question now changes from, What is God's purpose in miracles, and how should man respond? to, What exactly is the nature of the divine intervention in a miraculous event? The sign-value of miracle comes to be ignored; the main weight is on the transcendence of God's act of power.

St Thomas acknowledges the two-fold aspect of miracle:

> In miracles two aspects can be noted: one is what happens, something exceeding the normal bounds of nature, and because of this they are called miracles or acts of power (*miracula, virtutes*); the other is the reason why miracles happen, for the revealing of something supernatural, and because of this they are commonly called signs (*signa*). In short, on account of their excellence they are called wonders or marvels as if pointing to something far off (*Summa Theol*, IIa, q 178, q 1 ad 1).

But Père Monden, a leading Roman Catholic scholar, is severe in his judgment on the inadequacy of St Thomas' treatment of miracle—

> This definition takes note only of power as its characteristic; the fact of its being a sign seems to be an appendage added from outside; while it is certain that a miracle is caused by God, it is we who make of it a sign by our reasoning. The Biblical awareness of an intervention which God himself intends to be sign-bearing, is practically abandoned. This emasculated concept is to dominate theology and apologetic right up to the end of the nineteenth century. In periods contaminated by rationalism the breach between power and functional sign will be still further enlarged (*33, 50*).

The narrow, evidentialist, almost mechanical, reduction of miracle by St Thomas is quite explicit in another passage:

> Miracles lessen the merit of faith to the extent that they argue an unwillingness to believe the Scriptures, a hardness of heart that demands signs and wonders. All the

same, it is better for men to turn to the faith because of miracles than to remain altogether in their unbelief (*Summa Theol.*, IIIa, q 43, ad 2).

Monden rightly judges this concept of transcendence to be narrower than the fullness of tradition.

The medieval world-view broke up under the impact of men of science, in the first place astronomers—Galileo, Kepler and Newton; we may date it from about 1540 when Copernicus' *De Revolutionibus Orbium Celestium* was published. They led a revolt from the straight-jacket of medieval scholasticism, prizing above all the unfettered observation, plotting, and correlation of objects as they behave. The Schoolmen talked in terms of substance and essence, matter and form; the new thinkers were more interested in space and time, mass and energy. More important, they thought that their metaphysics was the last word, for they supposed that they could reduce the whole universe to basic particles of solid matter existing without purpose or beauty. This way of looking at the world was first accurately plotted by Descartes. His material world could be wholly reduced to mathematical terms. The minds of men were something quite different; and God had to be introduced to link the two together, and provide the laws which govern the material world. With such mental equipment modern science set out on its adventurous journey, and the equipment served up to the nineteenth century, the heyday of scientific materialism.

The first, and classic, assault on Christian miracles in the light of the new thinking, was made by Spinoza in his *Tractatus Theologico-Politicus*, of 1670. He assumes that science, and especially mathematics, is the key to understanding the universe, and most modern men who think at all about miracles would find themselves very much in sympathy with him. The ordinary person, says Spinoza, sees the unusual as the special sphere of God's activity, and assumes that God is inactive when nature proceeds naturally. (The phrase 'act of God' in insurance policies, referring to some dire and extreme emergency, still bears witness to this vulgar misinterpretation.) If God were to intervene, there would be two powers at work, the power of God and the power of nature: but this is impossible, because the laws of nature derive from the perfect nature of God, and those laws are eternal, fixed, and immutable. God cannot contradict himself, and so cannot 'intervene'. An irregularity in the course of nature could not possibly tell us anything about God; it could only make us doubt the existence of God.

Spinoza observed, rightly, that the Bible frequently assigns directly to God events which can be described in terms of nature's routine, and he deals drastically with the miracles in squeezing them into his chosen terms. He is alive also to the difficulties of historical certainty, and insists that we must know about the opinions of those who witnessed the miracles and also of those who wrote about them, and make a clear distinction between the event itself and the impression it may have made on the minds of the observers.

Here lie the seeds of all subsequent debate about miracles —historical, scientific, philosophical, and religious. We may at least be grateful to Spinoza for stating the terms of the debate so clearly.

John Locke was a man deeply concerned for the Christian gospel and equally concerned for the reign of reason, as may be gauged from the title of his work published in 1695, *The Reasonableness of Christianity*. For Locke, the existence of a God was an eminently reasonable belief; this could be reached by the mind's natural faculties. Faith, however, was demanded for

> the assent to any proposition, not thus made out by the deductions of reason, but upon the credit of the proposer, as coming from God in some extraordinary way of communication. This way of discovering truths to men we call *'revelation'*. (*An Essay Concerning Human Understanding,* Bk. 4, Ch. 18.2).

The question arises, how do we assess the 'credit of the proposer'? How does reason cope with the tests of prophecy-fulfilments and miracles? For Locke the fulfilment of prophecy was the success of a prediction. The Messiah had long been predicted, and with the appearance of Jesus of Nazareth the description fitted. This can be understood in a rather mechanical way, but Locke may have had in mind a deeper intuitive disclosure. Such intuition he certainly demands in the understanding of a miracle.

> A miracle then I take to be a sensible operation, which, being above the comprehension of the spectator, and in his opinion contrary to the established course of nature, is taken by him to be divine (*A Discourse of Miracles,* Introd.).

Miracles are God's credentials. But how shall we be sure that in any particular situation it is God's power which is displayed? A miracle must not be irreligious or immoral or trivial, and must relate to the glory of God and some great concern for men. In the end, Locke's estimate of miracles is not purely subjective: it is the divine power in miracles which is significant for him, and in trying to assess this he runs into the same difficulty as in his assessment of power in people. It is not exactly like civil power which can be

analysed into fines, prisons and so on. It does not fit wholly
into his categories of 'idea particulars'. It calls for an intuitive recognition. Belief in a powerful miracle is parallel to
belief in a powerful personality. From such a position it is
possible to maintain both the reasonableness and the mystery
of the Christian faith.

Locke's approach is particularly relevant to our contemporary situation. He was the founder of eighteenth-
century empiricism, and most philosophers today are
nothing if not empirical in their approach. Locke stoutly
maintained that there was no quarrel between reason and
revelation—a claim that many modern theologians would
do well to take seriously—but that this does not mean
reducing religion to fit a Procrustean bed of fashionable
physics.

The English Deists, men like Tindal and Toland, were
drastic in their treatment of Christian doctrine. They saw no
place for any divine revelation at all. God had given all men
perfect law by which to live and sufficient means to know it
and do it; so any special revelation by God is unnecessary,
and that recorded in the Bible is at many points unworthy of
the Deity. Thus miracles are doubly unnecessary.

Bishop Butler's answer in the *Analogy of Religion* (1736) is
as calm and meticulous as his opponents' case was wild and
frenzied. Regarding miracles, Butler is very much less
confident about the comprehensiveness of general laws of
nature:

> We are in such total darkness upon what causes,
> occasions, reasons, or circumstances, the present course of
> nature depends, that there does not appear any im-
> probability for or against supposing that five or six

thousand years may have given scope for causes from whence miraculous interpositions may have arisen,

particularly as he claimed to see

distinct particular reasons for miracles: to afford mankind instruction additional to that of nature, and to attest the truth of it.

For Butler miracles remain a major problem, because they seem to violate the congruity he is concerned to find between natural and revealed religion.

There was, however, a fundamental weakness which bedevilled both sides in the Deistic controversy. It was generally assumed that the method of apprehending Divine truth was the reasoned acceptance of intellectual propositions, and so it followed that revelation was concerned with the laws of nature, the means by which God arranges the reconciliation of sinners, and the terms required, backed by rewards and punishments. Much was spoken about the knowledge of things concerning God, but very little about any personal knowledge of God himself. It is hardly surprising that the level of ethics fell far below that of the New Testament. Lecky's description of the system as 'a theology which regarded Christianity as an admirable auxiliary to the police-force' is not unjustified.

The Deistic controversy did, however, have much more serious consequences in a different direction. The Deists, by fostering an empirical discussion of miracles, set about a radical attack on the historical reliability of the Christian revelation. The Deistic arguments may have been answered for the time being adequately by the orthodox, but the questioning of the literal infallibility of the Bible on rational grounds was going to have alarming consequences in a century's time. Already in 1683 Charles Blount had published a translation of the first two books of Philostratus' *Life of Apollonius of Tyana* with the intention of illustrating how miracles grow round the memory of eminent religious personages. In 1727 Anthony Collins propounded the view that the prophetic writings referred primarily to events in the lifetime of the prophets, including such passages as 'A virgin shall conceive...' From 1727 to 1729 appeared six discourses on miracles from Thomas Woolston, a Cambridge don of decidedly unstable mental condition, who contended that the Resurrection was a monstrous fraud engineered by the disciples who stole the body of Christ from the sepulchre. Woolston was charged with blasphemy and passed the last four years of his life in prison. As yet, and for many years, the church had no critical equipment with which to fight this battle.

A more serious work which focused current controversy to burning point was Hume's *Enquiry Concerning Human Understanding*, published in 1748. He starts by making a general attack on the reliability of human testimony. But there is for him a wider and more general difficulty. He sees no necessary connexion between natural events; their probability can only be reckoned by the number of times certain events have come together. So what is most likely is uniform, routine experience, and miracles are ruled out of court as altogether improbable from the nature of the case since they are bound to conflict with nature, and in this conflict lies their improbability.

A miracle is a violation of the laws of nature; and as a firm and unalterable experience has established these laws, the proof against a miracle, from the very nature of the fact, is as entire as any argument from experience can possibly be imagined.

E

Such an argument goes against Hume's own contention elsewhere that we can know nothing directly of laws and causes in nature, for in that case, if connexions do not exist between events, extraordinary events cannot be ruled out. Later Hume grants that in certain circumstances testimony may justify belief in something which 'seems' miraculous, though it cannot prove such an event to have been worked by God. Similarly a miracle can never be proved so certainly as to be the foundation of a particular system of religion. His essay certainly does not destroy belief in miracles, but it did serve to undermine the eighteenth-century view of miracles as an independent support for the truth of religion, and it raised, for the first time explicitly, difficulties connected with notions like 'violating the laws of nature' in a scientific context. Indirectly it did the Christian cause a service by forcing theologians to examine much more carefully what is implied in understanding and accepting the historical claims of Christian revelation.

Hume was not short of opponents. Of these we may take as typical Paley whose *Evidences of Christianity*, published in 1794, was required reading for entrants to the University of Cambridge up to the First World War.

Paley contends, with justice, that Hume had divorced miracles from their context, personal and moral. Miracles are not nearly as incredible as the life after death, an idea readily accepted in the natural theology which many Deists held. Any argument of miracles being 'contrary to general experience' is but a begging of the question. In any event, miracles were intended for the first launching of Christianity, and not to be much repeated after that. Above all, if twelve trusted men die to witness their belief in a miracle, is not this a powerful evidence for its truth? Later in his book

(Part 1, Ch. 9) Paley argues well the primitive character of the four gospels, evaluating our possession of genuine ancient manuscripts, their incorporation in the church's canon and liturgy, their ancient translation, and their use by the early Fathers and in ancient harmonies and commentaries. Here Paley leans upon evidences external to the New Testament, and here we may see the beginnings of modern New Testament scholarship, to which Paley himself contributed a useful study of correlations between *Acts* and the *Epistles of St Paul*. One of his contemporaries, Herbert Marsh, was already engaged upon an enquiry into the formation of the gospels.

In 1727 there died François de Paris, and at his tomb the Jansenists claimed a great number of miraculous cures. This sparked off considerable controversy about the miracles of saints, and Paley draws up a detailed system of canons to test the veracity of such reports. How far in time and distance are the reports from the events? How permanent has the belief been and how well confirmed from other sources? What effects did the miracles produce? Are the miracles simply a love of the marvellous, and do they simply bolster up already held beliefs? Was the perception of the miracles itself false? Was the miracle but one single success out of many attempts (like the King's Touch)? Was the cure merely of a nervous complaint? Has the transmission of the story itself changed an event into a miracle?

These are sound questions—and why should they not be asked of the Biblical miracles as well? Paley admits that some of the New Testament miracles would be disqualified by his canons, but claims that, taken together as a body they are beyond the reach of criticism. This historical critique, now directed to the study of the Bible itself, formed the seed-bed for later schools of constructive criticism which flowered in the work of Lightfoot, Westcott and Hort.

Today Paley's *Evidences* seems a very unsatisfactory book. His whole approach to Christian persuasion, which may be called evidentialism, is unprofitable. His concept of theology was too cut and dried. He supposed that 'natural theology' could give convincing reasons for the existence of God, and that miracles then provided a supernatural 'extra' to prove the revelation of God in Christ. Such a criticism does not despise the claims of natural theology (as they are widely despised in continental Protestant theology today): but it sees natural theology giving tentative pointers towards the Christian Creator God, and revealed theology offering significant clues towards the deep problems of man, his nature and his human predicament.

The evidentialists supposed that the truth of a miracle could be established purely by objective criteria, without need for any religious intuition or evaluation. This landed them in an impossible position because they observed only half of the definition of a miracle.

Further, they were far too confident about knowing the bounds of 'natural law'. It can be argued that if it were one day discovered that the faculties which enabled the Lord to do miracles can also belong to man, it would in no way affect his uniqueness; but such an argument would have been impossible to Paley and his followers.

In its simplest terms the evidentialist argument from miracles is circular, and therefore self-defeating—the fact that Christ did miracles proves that he was divine; whereas the miracle-stories are trustworthy because their author was divine.

To break this impasse an entirely new ingredient was needed, and it was supplied by one who is not usually thought of as being over-important for either theology or philosophy, John Wesley, who died in 1791, three years before the appearance of Paley's *Evidences*.

The philosophers of the Enlightenment, taking their cue from Descartes' *Cogito, ergo sum*—'I think, therefore I am'—had valued the mind and its reasoning processes as highly as they had undervalued emotion and intuition in the matter of religion. After all most people, if they paused to seek a good reason for believing that they were people, would answer not 'I think', but 'I feel'—love or hate, joy or sorrow, pain or pleasure. Against Descartes' rarefied view of human nature, human nature now made its protest—a very vociferous protest—in the Evangelical Revival.

Wesley's dramatic preaching called for, and called forth, an inward conviction resulting in a new life of reconciliation with Christ. Christian certitude was now an internal assurance, a veritable new birth, based on a value-judgment of the gospel story made by heart and soul as well as mind; a process far removed from intellectual assent to external evidences.

This is not to say that Wesley discounted the facts of history. He had full faith in the miracles of Christ and of the church of the first three centuries. He also expected miracles in answer to prayer, but he would examine any particular record of one very critically. The idea of a general providence without a particular providence was for him nonsense. But the new signs of the spirit were more convincing evidence than the testimony of the gospel miracles. Faith was nothing less than the power of God working within us to enable us to see through the world of visible things to that world which is invisible and eternal. Regeneration rather than illumination was now the criterion of spiritual reality.

From a very different starting-point the Oxford

Movement shared with the Evangelical Movement a rediscovery of the proper place of emotion and intuition in the
religious life, as it shared also its belief in the literal inspiration of the Bible. Both movements between them provided
a providential deliverance from the aridities of eighteenth-
century thought and prepared Christians for the later-
nineteenth-century critical onslaught on the text and context
of the Bible itself.

If Wesley and the evangelicals erred too far in their
emphasis on the personal and subjective element in faith,
the balance was corrected by S. T. Coleridge, a thinker
whose contribution has been underestimated, for he exer-
cised a deep influence on such different personalities as J. H.
Newman and F. D. Maurice. Personal and subjective response was for him of vital importance. In his *Confessions
of an Enquiring Spirit* (1840) he protests against the tyranny of
literal inspiration of the Bible, and sees inspiration in the
fact that the Bible 'finds me' at a far greater depth than all
other books put together. But he was not interested in
religious ideas, any more than the Bible is interested in
religious ideas. He was interested in the facts (or acts) of
Christ's incarnation and redemption. The foundation of his
faith was:

> the belief that a means of salvation has been effected and
> provided for the human race by the incarnation of the
> Son of God in the person of Jesus Christ; and that his
> life on earth, his sufferings, death and resurrection are
> not only proofs and manifestations, but likewise essential
> and effective parts of the great redemptive act (*Aids to
> Reflection*, 1884 ed., p. 130).

In miracle we have the union of objective fact with subjective faith, for as he observed, 'miracles could open the

eyes of the body; and he that was born blind beheld his
redeemer. But miracles, even those of the Redeemer himself,
could not open the eyes of the self-blinded' (*Confessions*,
1849 ed., p. 78).

Coleridge rightly resorts to scripture itself to support his
assertion that miracles by themselves cannot work a true
conviction of the mind. Those who reject inward spiritual
truth will not be persuaded though one rose from the
dead:

> Is it not that implication of doctrine in the miracle and
> of miracle in the doctrine, which is the bridge of com-
> munication between the senses and the soul? (*The
> Friend*, 1863 ed., II, ii, p. 144).

Coleridge maintained a loyalty to a fully incarnational
theology, coupled equally with a sensitive insight into the
personal nature of faith which is an object-lesson for today.

By the middle of the nineteenth century the full blast of
radical German criticism of the New Testament had reached
this country, principally in the two-volume *Life of Jesus* by
D. F. Strauss, translated by George Eliot. Here Strauss
'demythologises' with a vengeance. In the matter of miracles
this is his canon of judgment:

> If the particular nature of an event not only is suspect
> in the eyes of criticism and its external 'ornamentation'
> exaggerated etc., but also if its inner core and foundation
> are either inconceivable or display a striking resemblance
> to the Messianic conceptions of the Jews of that time, not
> only the given 'facts' of the matter but the whole event
> as such must be regarded as unhistorical.

Strauss's intention is to reduce Jesus to 'proper' historical
size and to credit St Paul and the early church with having

inflated him to a mythical Christ. Following Hegel, however, Strauss maintains that the inner core of his Christian
faith is completely independent of his critical research:

> Christ's natural birth, his miracles, his resurrection and
> ascension, these remain eternal truths, however greatly
> their reality as historical facts is to be doubted.

There seems to be a strong family likeness between Strauss
and Bultmann!

Fortunately, to meet this German invasion, England was
able to produce the trio of great Cambridge scholars,
Westcott, Lightfoot and Hort. But this time in the matter of
the historicity of miracles, Christian apologists were on the
defensive. Up to 1850 the reliability of the miracle accounts
had not been seriously called in question. Then the miracles,
instead of proving the truth of the gospel, became a
positive hindrance to its credibility.

How did they conduct their defensive campaign? They
introduced the argument, a familiar one today, that the
miracles are too integral a part of the historical life of
Christ to be cut out altogether: if that is done, the fragments
which remain are of no worth. Westcott emphasises the
human setting of the miracles, especially the great personal
effort which they cost the Lord, and the element of human
faith which often seems to condition their response. Miracles
are, for Westcott,

> all faint reflections of the glory of the Incarnation. That is
> the miracle of miracles to which all others point (*Charac-
> teristics of the Gospel Miracles*, 1859, p. 3).

They are the treasure, rather than the bulwark, of the faith.

> In meaning, as well as in time, they lie between the
> Incarnation and the Ascension: they look back to the
> coming of God to man, and forward to the bringing of

man to God. They become an evidence of his faith to a Christian who understands them rightly (*Characteristics*, p. 7).

In trying to extract the fullest spiritual meaning from each miracle, however, Westcott enters the dangerous territory of allegory. The stilling of the storm, for example, bears the heading 'The defence of the church from without'. Westcott finds three classes of healing miracles: those brought about by the faith of the sufferer, those by the mediation of friends, and those by the spontaneous mercy of Christ; from which we have lessons in faith, intercession, and love. This is perilously near reading meaning into events rather than out of them.

It was however a real discovery of nineteenth-century theology that miracle may be God's unique sign-language to us, and Westcott insists that such personal dealing with us by God is always subtle. Those who see the event but fail to see the sign are at liberty to describe or explain the event in other terms. It required courage thus to demolish the evidentialist structure of apologetic which had been one of the main bastions of the church for centuries.

A further complication for the Christian apologist came from the side of science in the person of T. H. Huxley, well known for his popularisation of scientific ideas and for his controversy with Christian leaders, the most familiar being his successful skirmish with Bishop Wilberforce in 1862 at the British Association. The main difficulty about miracles for the scientist, says Huxley, is not the uniformity of nature, but the credibility of evidence. The more unusual the event, the better the evidence required for believing it. It is notable that here Huxley is arguing on the grounds not of science but of history. 'Scientific' history was as yet young, and in his day had modelled itself closely on the principles of the physical sciences, but we may conclude that Huxley was a better scientist than he was historian.

Concerning nature he was quite definite. In his life of David Hume (published in 1879) he says that to define a miracle, as Hume did, as a 'violation of the laws of nature' was an employment of language which could not be justified. If a dead man did come to life, this would indicate not a breaking of any law of nature, but a proving it to be inadequate. But Huxley also maintained that there is no sufficient evidence for believing any one particular miracle in the Bible.

This frank admission from the side of science that the boundaries of scientific knowledge are not clearly defined was at first greeted with joy by the theologians, for now no miracle could be proved impossible. But their joy was turned to consternation when they realised that if the natural could not be defined, neither could the supernatural. Any talk of 'divine intervention' was now impossible. How then could a miracle be recognised? This threw the apologists right back on to the sign-value of miracle, and marked the final dissolution of the evidentialist approach. The understanding of the New Testament miracles is from now on inextricably bound up with the understanding of the whole New Testament witness to Jesus Christ. For this deliverance Christians may be profoundly glad.

The period of the Darwinian controversy, just one hundred years ago, tends to be recorded in history books in terms of absolute and uncomprehending opposition on the part of Christian leaders. This is far from the truth. Frederick Temple (later Archbishop of Canterbury) in his book *The Relations between Religion and Science,* published in 1884, welcomed the theory of organic evolution as enriching

Paley's argument that discovering a watch must lead on to belief in a watchmaker. By this time the leading Christian thinkers clearly understood that the scientific method dealt with abstractions drawn from generalisations, and so at best could only offer an incomplete picture of things. Temple denied that there is a science of physics comparable in precision with mathematics and sharing its logic, and refused to allow that all events could be fully explained by the principle of physics.

This claim became the harder to make because history also was being modelled on physical 'laws'. But to reduce all events to a mechanical process of cause and effect is to leave out the one indubitable factor in human activity, the exercise of free-will, and indeed free-will provides the best human analogy for the sphere of the miraculous. If 'nature' is to include the nature of God, immanent as well as transcendent, then to make a claim for miracle is to make a 'free-will' claim for the universe. The theologians very properly contended for a theological use of words like 'nature', 'cause,' and 'law', as well as a scientific use.

F. Temple wrote, 'If a miracle were worked, science could not prove that it was a miracle, nor of course prove that it was not a miracle.' And again, it is possible that 'the intervention which has apparently disturbed the sequence of phenomena is, after all, that of a higher physical law as yet unknown'. Temple gave as an example faith-healing, the strange power of mind over body, about which little was then known (psychology being an infant science) but, for all that, probably falling within the realm of science. It was realised that on this argument Christ's miracles of healing might turn out not to be miraculous (in one particular sense). They could still remain evidence of the compassion of the Son of Man.

This radically new approach of the Victorians demanded an overall congruity of purpose or value. If miracles were to be distinctive of revelation, this is not because they were different from human experience; it must be because they signified and symbolised man's highest ideals and aspirations. Only so could they possibly be expressions of the divine free-will.

The impressive figure of Charles Gore not only linked the nineteenth and twentieth centuries, but also linked Biblical criticism, divine immanence and organic evolution with the traditional doctrine of the church—no mean feat! Gore accepted the oral tradition underlying the gospels, and insisted on maintaining the miraculous stories, because if these could not be trusted, the recorded word of the Lord could be trusted even less. Gore struggled hard and long to maintain (against modernists and liberals) that the Christian revelation *was* a particular series of acts of God in history, some of which were miraculous in the full sense of that word, and not a set of ideas or truths connected with them.

Setting these particular acts of God within the context of history and nature, Gore contends, in the Bampton Lectures of 1891, that this supernatural act of God in Christ is the natural climax to the process of evolution. Evolution is the record of progress from the inorganic to the personal, and the person of Christ alone reveals in full the love and righteousness of the Creator. To Christ, representing a new level in creation, miracles are natural. Christ came not to teach men about salvation, but to save them, and his miracles are part of his restoration of the true order of nature.

By the 1930s a very different picture of the universe was being drawn by the scientists themselves, and thinkers like

A. N. Whitehead were speaking of it not as a collection of static things, but rather as a process of an infinite variety of events. From this vastly more complex view of the world it must be concluded that scientific investigation can never give an exhaustive account of any one situation, even in its physical aspect. The scientific method can never be the key to all reality.

H. H. Farmer elaborates this theme in his book *The World and God* (1935) and warns us against too uniform an idea of the world. He prefers a pluralistic view, the interplay of a great number of lower created agents, while persons are created creators, standing in personal relationship with the eternal personal. God's activity will then be at two levels: directly with sub-personal entities, using their ordinary routine; but, with people, in a way that does not overrule their personal will. Even if there is no co-operation, they can still be used as unwitting agents of his purpose.

This kind of picture is probably unfamiliar to many people (for much popular Christian apologetic has hardly moved out of the eighteenth century), and so it calls for some elaboration.

4. The Logical Placing of Miracle

DR JOHNSON is supposed once to have passed two washer-women shouting at each other across the street from opposite houses and remarked that they would never agree because they were arguing from different premises. Even a cursory survey of the relations between science and religion in the last hundred years illustrates a good deal of similar confusion arising because the logical status of the terms used had not been clarified. Many of the scientists assumed that there was only one logical pattern of thought—the scientific one —and some of the less circumspect Christian apologists played into their hands by sharing this unargued pre-supposition. Some eminent Victorian scientists showed incredible naivety in transferring their scientific methods, often grossly over-simplified, into the realm of religion. Edmund Gosse relates in that delightful but frightening autobiography of his childhood, *Father and Son*, how his father, Sir Philip Gosse, F.R.S., the eminent marine biologist,

> retained the singular superstition, amazing in a man of scientific knowledge and long human experience, that all pains and ailments were directly sent by the Lord in chastisement for some definite fault, and not in relation to any physical cause. The result was sometimes quite startling, and in particular I recollect that my stepmother and I exchanged impressions of astonishment at my father's action when Mrs. Goodyer, who was one of the

'Saints' and the wife of a young journeyman cobbler, broke her leg. My father, puzzled for an instant as to the meaning of this accident, since Mrs. Goodyer was the gentlest and most inoffensive of our church members, decided that it must be because she had made an idol of her husband, and he reduced the poor thing to tears by standing at her bed-side and imploring the Holy Spirit to bring this sin home to her conscience (*Father and Son*, 1913 ed., p. 273).

We live today in an empirical world. Philosophers want to know what actually is the case, and how it can be verified in experience. For any verbal bills of exchange philosophers want to be assured of cash value. Christians need not be alarmed at this, for the incarnation represents just such a claim—that the creator-God expressed himself in terms 'which we have heard, which we have seen with our eyes, which we have looked upon, and our hands have handled ...' (I John 1.1). So the task of metaphysics is not to reveal hidden mysteries but to make coherent sense of the whole of human experience, which includes creeds and canticles as well as microbes and mesons.

In the last three centuries discoveries in the physical sciences have changed the face of the earth and man's whole manner of life to an unprecedented degree. Popular opinion tends to suppose that the only pure and accurate account of things will be given in terms used in the laboratory, where natural laws are formulated which never shall be broken. In fact, nothing of the sort happens in a laboratory. Scientists first choose what small section of the natural order they want to observe, then from their observations they produce a generalisation. Water is boiled a hundred times and its temperature measured, and it is discovered that, on the whole, the boiling point is 100°C. One feature has been abstracted from the situation and generalised into a hypothesis, with the strong expectation and prediction that, next time water is boiled, the result will again be 100°C. If, however, the experiment is repeated at the top of a mountain or at the bottom of a coal mine, the result will not be 100°C. The scientist re-examines his hypothesis and finds that he has omitted an important qualification concerning atmospheric pressure, and then all is well. Until he enters the sub-atomic field and is compelled now to talk in terms of 'heavy water', whose behaviour is very different from H_2O. To cover this and other relevant statements he will need to produce a new hypothesis concerning the nature and motion of the constituent elements.

As he progresses, he comes up against an event or fact that seems to be relevant, but does not fit in with the existing hypothesis. At first he digs his heels in, checks the accuracy of his working, doubts the blighter's relevance, but since he is committed to seeking ever more comprehensive schemes of uniformity, he is eventually compelled to include the newcomer, even if it means reshaping the whole hypothesis.

From this kind of procedure two facts emerge which are vital in any assessment of scientific statements. In the first place, every scientific statement concerns an abstraction, something less than the totality of the original concrete item. The more comprehensive the abstract generalisation, the farther removed it is from the concrete original. The more it professes to tell, the less it can tell about. In the second place, every scientific statement is incomplete, or science would grind to a halt. Scientific enquiry progresses and develops by building on the inadequacies of past generalisations. There is no reason to suppose that this will stop, for there is no limit to the divisibility of space-time; but at the bounds of infinitely asking the question, Why is ...? the scientist will end up with such a question as, Why is there anything at all?—and the answering of that lies outside the field of scientific method.

It must be clear then that the categories of science cannot cope with miracle, which is by definition a non-conforming event. If a miracle happened in a laboratory, as Frederick Temple perceived, the scientific observer, *qua* scientist, could only say, 'Here's a queer thing!'; but he could prove neither that it was a miracle nor that it was not a miracle. If he were a keen scientist one would hope he would go on to try to incorporate this event into a wider uniformity, but this would take him outside the laboratory. To talk of laws of nature being broken (or not broken) is just nonsense: 'breaking' does not apply to laws which are only tentative formulations of generalised abstractions. If the miracles of the Bible are squeezed to fit into scientific-type talk, we are left with the five thousand sharing hidden packets of sandwiches, the rebuke to the storm being really directed to the disciples, and healing miracles as acts of hypnotic suggestion.

In short, to talk of God's making laws or God's breaking them is misleading because it puts 'God' into the category of a scientific hypothesis, which he is not. Laplace, the astronomer, was logically justified when, in answer to Napoleon's asking him where he fitted God in to his Newtonian scheme of the universe, he replied, 'I have no need of that hypothesis'. 'Of course you can't fit God into the picture:' protested Dean Inge, 'he is the canvas on which the picture is painted'.

If God cannot be comprehended by scientific language,

F

is there any other sort of language which can contain 'miracle'? If science is a language of abstract generalisation based on observed fact, is there a language dealing with life at a more concrete level which would serve better? Let us try history.

> The Art of Biography
> Is different from Geography.
> Geography is about Maps,
> But Biography is about Chaps.

We may seize on this useful distinction of E. C. Bentley's, and extend his dictum about biography to include history. Economic historians may claim that history is about profit and capital and labour; political historians read or write history in terms of kings and commons and constitutions, but basically history is about people. The historian chooses a person or event or cluster of people or events which he judges to be important, and tries to re-present them in their historical setting in such a way that his reader may see the relevance of such a personal encounter for his own time and place.

Unlike science, which seeks the truth in uniformities derived from abstractions, history seeks the truth in relevancies drawn from concretions. The purest history is that of maximum concreteness.

I. T. Ramsey likens the two sorts of quest to someone trying to penetrate the life of a Norfolk village (*38*, 10). He could arm himself with a map which would give him a precise knowledge of certain features of the village, remembering that the sheet which covers the largest area gives the fewest details. Such is the scientific method. Or he could go and talk with the village postmaster or police-man (assuming that they had lived there some time), and in this personal encounter he could come face to face, as it were, with the living heart of the place. Such a picture, built up from many and varied personal impressions, would be of the maximum concreteness.

The notion of history as a 'scientific' means of establishing the truth is a fairly modern one—no earlier than the nineteenth century—and since historians then were much influenced by the pretensions of science, they too have sometimes claimed more than their due. G. F. Woods has made quite plain in his lecture *Contemporary Theological Liberalism* (*62*, 5) that there is no such thing as a neutral historical method which is devoid of presuppositions about the structure and working of the world. Especially where the evidence is thin, historians inevitably tend to read into their reconstruction of events what they think must have happened.

> The unavoidable presence of presuppositions in the making of historical enquiries means that there is no metaphysically uncommitted bar of history to which appeal can be made. Final verdicts are not attainable in a court which does not administer the same law in all cases and where the procedures are so diverse. The quest for an empirical method quite free from any metaphysical presumptions is a vain quest.

So, then, from the point of view of history also, we are thrown back on to metaphysics. If ever we are to achieve one method of discourse, one 'language map' to cover the whole of human experience we need certain key metaphysical words. They are necessary for science to draw together its various disparate branches, to unite them into a common field, and to raise to a level of concreteness what in science is abstracted. They are necessary in history to provide a criterion for selection and extension. We are claiming that the 'top' key words of metaphysics are 'I' and 'God', for these alone can be used at any and every level of language because they belong to none. They are also the terms of maximum concreteness.

The total territory to be mapped in any world-view must include ourselves, and our whole selves at that. But in trying to describe ourselves we run into difficulty. I observe myself to be—all sorts of things; and my friends (and foes) who observe me could add a good deal more. But when every sort of objective analysis of 'me' has been made, 'I' remain something over and above statements about 'me'. 'I' in my concreteness am more than the sum of all statements that can be made about me—or that I can make about myself. In fact, I am I, which may be tautological but is not nonsensical because it points to the peculiar logic necessary for dealing with persons. Objective statements about 'me' become public property, as can all the results of sense-perceptions; yet at heart I retain a quality of 'I-ness' which can never become public property. The French, with sensitive logic, have two different words for 'knowing'— *savoir*, to know inferentially, to know things, to know that, and, significantly, to know how; and *connaître*, the non-inferential knowledge of persons, a concrete awareness.

Much of the work of science consists of pinning things down and labelling them. The labelling of persons, however, is not so straightforward. Primitive peoples, as also the Hebrews of the Old Testament, have a great reluctance to disclose their names because they feel that to know a person's name is to know something important of his nature, and so to be a way of acquiring power over him. Coming up to Norwich in the train a little time ago I sat opposite a United States serviceman and observed that he wore his name for all to read on a name-plate sewn on to his tunic. I felt that this was an intolerable invasion of his private life. Most of us wear various labels, of varying degrees of abstraction. 'The Brigadier' (most abstract); William Fitz-Maurice (less abstract); Bill, to his friends, and Bimbo to his intimates (in greater degrees of concreteness). Each works on a different level of awareness, and the most concrete of all presents us with a disclosure situation in depth. 'Peter answereth and saith unto him, Thou art the Christ' (Mk 8.29). 'Jesus saith unto her, Mary. She turned herself, and saith unto him, Rabboni; which is to say, Master' (Jn 20.16). 'Thomas answered and saith unto him, My Lord and my God' (Jn 20.28).

Which brings us back to miracles. A miracle is a disclosure-event. Like any other event it can be analysed objectively, but to do so is to miss the point, to side-step the disclosure. In the logic of language, to see a miracle is more akin to seeing a joke than to seeing a red omnibus, and the more you analyse a joke, the less of a joke does it become. Plenty of people saw the wonders, the non-conforming events of Jesus, but few saw their point; and our records tell us that, logically enough, Jesus refused to do miracles where there was no likelihood of their point being grasped. They would not only *not* disclose the mystery, but would positively put people on to the wrong track. Hence the standing lament of the prophets, 'By hearing ye shall hear, and shall not understand; and seeing ye see, and shall not perceive; for this people's heart is waxed gross, and their ears are dull of hearing, and their eyes they have closed; lest at any time they should see with their eyes, and hear with their ears, and should understand with their heart, and should be converted, and I should heal them' (Mt 13.14–15, quoted from Is 6.9–10).

From the point of view of history, then, a miracle is an

event of peculiar significance and special relevance. It is a disclosure-situation which can only adequately be described by reference to the activity of God. (Much the same could be said for the parables.)

But miracles are more; they are events which do not conform with the normal pattern: they attract people's attention by their strangeness. How does God fit in to this linguistic landscape? Such a metaphysical term as 'God' is necessary, we have said, to give unity and concreteness to the various scientific languages. (This makes an act of faith that the universe is a unity, which most scientists and philosophers are happy to subscribe to, even if they do not care for the term 'God'.) This is really a restatement of the classical ontological argument for the existence of God.

But within this unity which is established by God's active relatedness to all things, we must distinguish two kinds of activity. There is first of all his activity in the world of things—the 'laws' of nature—for whose explication the physical sciences provide the appropriate language (or languages). Theology will speak of God's general providence, and a religious scientist like the great botanist John Ray will be happy to entitle his book *The Wisdom of God in the Works of Creation*.

No less important, however, is God's activity in the world of persons (and we must not forget that the world of things and the world of persons add up to one world), for which the language of history is appropriate. The claim of miracle is just this: that in history we have seen in a particular set of events God's personal activity at work in a remarkable way.

Anyone who is asked the question, 'Do miracles happen?' should be guided by the Methodist minister who, when asked 'Can Methodists dance?' replied, 'Some can and some can't'. For the question is not a matter of law but a matter of history. The so-called conflict between science and miracles, as Ramsey insists, is a pseudo-conflict. The question 'Do miracles occur?' implies a science-language answer which is not appropriate. It must be turned to 'Did a particular miracle occur on such and such an occasion?', which demands a history-language answer, which is appropriate.

So the questioner must examine all the available and relevant evidence: in the case of New Testament miracles, this means a careful assessment of the documents, their history and background; a survey of the events which seem to have resulted from the miracles; and the witness contributed by the tradition of the church in creed and worship. He will be prepared to admit God's personal activity working oddly, that is, in the sub-personal world (in the case of nature miracles and perhaps in the case of healing miracles), realising that this breaks no laws, but reveals the pattern of God's activity to be more complex than is usually understood. He will have to ask whether the problem can be solved without introducing such an idea as 'God's personal activity'. And he will no doubt ask whether such a record is relevant only to past time or whether it speaks to our condition today.

He will find himself searching for a more adequate way of talking which will embrace both worlds, of things and of persons, into one scheme, and may find clues in logically complex words like 'activity'. He may very well realise that the result of his quest will not just be intellectual satisfaction but a challenge to his whole person which can only be answered by worship. Within the context of traditional Christian worship he will find that many have trodden this hard way before him, when for instance he hears St Paul write to the Colossians of the cosmic Christ in whom all

things are held together; or when he turns to the Order of
Morning Prayer and finds as alternative canticles the
Benedicite calling for every part of the natural creation to
give praise to its Creator, and the *Te Deum* giving glory to
God for his mighty works of redemption in history.

So much, then, by way of warning that the logical
background of the concept of miracle is not as straightforward as it might seem. It can never be fixed among the
terms and on the level of scientific discourse. It fits more
properly among the personal terms of historical discourse.
Even here we must beware of importing ideas of 'scientific' precision into historical judgments. Miracles, we
claim, are a particularly personal disclosure of God, and
they require a no less intimately personal appreciation.

To ignore or mistake the proper logical placing of
miracles is to invite a head-on collision between 'scientific'
medicine on the one hand and 'unscientific' religion on the
other. The next chapter must unhappily recount the course of
this conflict, or pseudo-conflict, as it developed over the
centuries, though it can end on a happier note with some
important signs of present-day reconciliation.

5. Religion and Medicine: The Story of a Pseudo-conflict

OUR subject is 'healing miracles', and so far we have not progressed much beyond 'miracles'. This long preliminary treatment has been necessary because the concept of 'miracle' is a complex one, and unless we have sorted out our premises, our argument will be as unprofitable as that of Dr Johnson's washerwomen.

Unfortunately the concept of 'healing' is not much simpler. It is easier to define sickness than health, and clearly an absence of symptoms is part of the story (though most healthy people have symptoms if there were opportunity to observe them). The World Health Organisation has a definition in terms of physical, mental and social well-being, and mental health authorities include the ability to cope with mental conflict, to work, and to love (*59, 37*). At least we must be sufficiently Hebraic to insist that 'health' include man and his relationships, and as we shall see there is a strong link between a person's relationships and the state of his physical well-being.

Some historical sketch of the relations between medicine and religion from Biblical times until now is required for two reasons. We must beware against importing modern ideas about medicine uncritically into a consideration of the New Testament miracles. And if those miracles have something to say to us today about health and healing, this must be set against today's picture (in so far as there is one), or again we shall be talking at cross-purposes. The first part of this chapter will attempt an analysis of the conflict or, rather, pseudo-conflict; the second part will sketch some factors which may make for a synthesis.

A. CONFLICT

The scientific study of medicine did not start with the Greeks. Ancient China, Egypt, and India had well-developed medical skills, but since our theme is principally a European one, we will start with the Greeks, those remarkable people whose world extended from the coast and islands of Asia Minor to Sicily and southern Italy. They were keen observers of life around them, and had a passionate desire to bring their observations into an intelligible wholeness. Heraclitus' dictum 'All things are in flux' witnesses to their sense of variety; Parmenides' watchword, 'Reality is the changeless' to their desire for unity. From the very first the medical workers defined health in terms of proportion or balance. Alcmaeon of Croton, the first Greek to write a medical treatise, to practise dissection, and to fix upon the brain as the centre of the sensory-motor system, declared '*isonomia* (balanced regulation) is health'. Upset balance he calls *monarchia*, and this is the cause of disease. There indeed is a remarkable anticipation of what Cannon in the early twentieth century labelled *homeostasis*, the body's ability to recover its physical balance after an upset. This deep conviction of a pervading balance or harmony, both in man and in the whole natural order, was fundamental to the Greek outlook and can be traced right down to Aristotle's ethics, the apotheosis of the doctrine of the 'golden mean'.

Empedocles (of Acragas, in Sicily) has won the title 'father of chemistry' from his formulation of the hypothesis that all things are constituted from the four basic elements of fire, air, water, and earth, a dogma which had one of the longest runs of any human authoritative pronouncement. It held sway until the arrival of phlogiston, and even in the seventeenth century the physiology of breathing required the concept of fire in the chest. The number four was invested with a near-mystical importance as, for example, the four temperaments which arose from the four humours associated with wet, dry, hot, and cold.

Hippocrates of Cos is rightly called the father of Greek medical science, though as with Solomon much wisdom was gathered under his name, and it is not easy to sort out what rightly belongs to him. But what does not is still a tribute to his influence. His life (c. 460–377 BC), spanning the great days of Greece, made him an older contemporary of Plato. He builds on Empedocles' doctrine of four elements; he shows a wide, but very critical, interest in the drugs in common use; he has a keen influence in the interest of environment and climate; he has a profound trust in the value of a sense of calmness and security in his patient, and also the sanctity of medical work.

He was also the first physician to be seriously concerned with psychological medicine. He recognised the brain as an organ of mind; he looked for a physiological explanation of emotional disorders; he pinned down the body fluids, phlegm and bile, as being responsible for emotional states (the word 'melancholy' still reflects his diagnosis of an excess of black bile); and he vigorously attacked the idea of illness as something divinely ordained. Epilepsy had for long been known as the sacred disease, and this made Hippocrates very angry; it was 'in no way more divine, or more sacred than any other diseases, but has a natural cause . . .' Of the 'purificators' who treated epilepsy by incantations he wrote, 'it seems to me, they make the divinity out to be most wicked and impious. ... Such persons thus use the divinity as a screen for their own inability to afford any assistance'. An awful warning against a 'god of the gaps'!

He seems to have been the first person to try to remove mental illness and its cure from the realm of philosopher and priest to that of objective study. Against this he encountered great opposition, and nearly a hundred and fifty years were to pass before another physician was bold enough to continue this side of his work. Plato himself re-opened the door to the notion of sacred and profane forms of madness, with disastrous results to follow in the Middle Ages.

Aristotle, the pupil of Plato and the son of a court physician (384–322 BC), ranks as the first real scientist we know. He had an almost divine faith in the power of human reason and a very wide and practical knowledge of biology. But he parted company with Hippocrates on many issues: for him the body fluids were merely conductors of heat and cold; he saw no connexion between the brain and psychological states except in so far that it condensed 'by means of its cold consistency, the hot vapours which arose from the heart, which vapours then formed a dew which fell and refreshed the heart, making it more temperate'. Which sounds very Victorian!

Greek history for schoolboys ends at 362 BC, but Greek science, and especially Greek medicine, did not. At Alexandria Hierophilus and Erasistratus developed the practice of dissection (upon the bodies of executed criminals), and studied the connexion of blood with the heart, and of nerves with the brain.

The principal contribution to mental science was made in the middle of the first century BC by Asclepiades, an orator turned physician. His writings are lost, but his life is recorded by Aurelian, one of the earliest medical historians. He had no time for the term 'insanity': it was a vulgar and unscientific description. He distinguished carefully fever-delirium from more chronic forms of mental illness, and delusions from hallucinations (a distinction more or less ignored until the nineteenth century). He located the cause of most mental illness in profound emotional disturbance and devised original treatment for his patients, condemning the usual dungeons and advocating instead such pleasant occupations as swinging hammocks and baths, music and harmony. He saw little difference between bleeding and strangling, though the former was to continue as standard treatment for fifteen centuries.

Aurelian himself was unable to share such liberal views, and was particularly distressed by sexual perversions. He wrote a book *De Incubone*, in which he lent the weight of his own authority to the prevalent view that there existed a demon, called an incubus, in form like a man, whose business it was to seduce women sexually and so gain control over their souls. The corresponding female demon was the succubus, an equal menace to men. In this doctrine lies the foundation of a demonology which for sixteen hundred years was to spell torture and death for hundreds of thousands of insane men and women.

The Classical period comes to a triumphant conclusion in the person of Galen, a physician from Pergamum, in Asia Minor, who had a brilliant medical career and a popular practice in Rome from 162 until his death in AD 199. He tried to preserve what was best in the Hippocratic tradition, choosing those aspects of current philosophical and religious thought which he found most acceptable. He has the distinction of being the first influential writer to stand up for

Christians, not being one himself, against their detractors, on philosophical grounds. (He was a great worshipper of the god Aesculapius who, he claimed, had cured him of a dangerous abscess.) In the course of practical experiments he established that pressure on the brain produced unconsciousness and paralysis, whereas pressure on the heart affected only the blood vessels, and so concluded that the brain, not the heart, is the seat of reason. He was within an ace of discovering the circulation of blood, but this had to wait until 1628 and William Harvey. On the other hand, his standard treatment for festering wounds and inflammations was *terra sigillata*, red clay compressed into round cakes and stamped with the image of the goddess Diana.

With the death of Galen the dark ages of medicine set in, and scientific progress marked time for well over a thousand years—from the third century to the seventeenth. Not only was there no progress, but in the matter of mental illness there was a tragic regression.

The attitude of the early Christian church to the practice of medicine was ambiguous. There was a strong feeling that Christian faith and prayer should be enough to work miracles of healing so that the doctor was unnecessary. Eusebius, the church historian, recounts the splendid martyr's death of two Christian doctors, Alexander of Phrygia, and Zenobius (*Historia Eccl.*, VIII. 13. 4), and praises Bishop Theodotus as being skilled in the healing of bodies and minds. Tatian (*c.* AD 160 *Oratio ad Graecos*, 20) allows medicine for the heathen, but not for Christians; St Ambrose disapproved of medicine and St Bernard of Clairvaux (AD 1090–1153) forbade it for his monks. Canon law laid down that medical instructions were in conflict with divine knowledge. Surgery had been discouraged by the Emperor Justinian (AD 527–567) who closed the medical schools of Athens and Alexandria. The *coup de grâce* was administered in AD 1215 by Pope Innocent III who condemned surgery and all priests practising it. In 1248 the dissection of the body was pronounced sacrilegious and the study of anatomy condemned.

Far more sinister was the rise, to a pathological degree, of a belief in demon-possession, and a weird flood of exorcism to counter it. It was universally assumed that mentally abnormal people were witches or inhabited by devils, and to seek out and kill such people became a religious duty on the authority of the commands in Exodus 22.18 and Leviticus 20.27. It had been forgotten, apparently, that a large part of Christ's earthly ministry had been spent in healing and helping such people. The first formal execution of a witch took place about AD 430, and how many thousands followed will never be known. In the reign of Francis I of France over one hundred thousand are said to have been killed. The Reformed Church was no better. In the year 1515 at Geneva five hundred were burnt at the stake in three months.

The classic document setting forth in hideous detail the reason for belief in witches and witchcraft, the signs by which they could be identified, and the full technique for torturing and burning them, is the *Malleus Maleficarum*, the *Hammer of the Witches*, prepared by two monks, Henry Kramer and James Sprenger, in accordance with a Papal Bull of 1484 for the purpose of purging Christendom of a great invasion of demons, witches, succubi, and incubi. A few brave medical men made their protest, Paracelsus, Juan Luis Vives, and Cornelius Agrippa of Nettesheim, the last of whom denounced the Inquisition, and died penniless, alone, and reviled.

A pupil of Agrippa's, Johann Weyer, having obtained a

secure position as personal physician to Duke William of
Jülich, risked a head-on clash with the Inquisition. He
assailed the current theories which 'prejudiced the life and
safety of medicine, the most ancient, the most useful, and
the most necessary of all sciences', and he exploded these
theories by a careful comparison of the symptoms of his
mentally ill patients with those given in the *Malleus Maleficarum* for the identification of witches. The confessions which
such people made were, he claimed, often symptoms of
their illness. This struggle by Weyer, himself a deeply
religious man, to bring mental illness out of the spheres
of law and religion into that of medicine, met with violent
reaction. Bodin, one of the leading lawyers of the Middle
Ages, attacked Weyer for doubting that witches ate babies'
flesh, and that women were particularly prone to sorcery and
witchcraft, being liars, having larger intestines than men,
and being half way between men and wild beasts.

Public opinion was slow to move. In England the laws
against witchcraft were not repealed until 1736.

During these dark centuries, scientific observation of
nature gave way to legend and allegory, fable and heraldry,
the phoenix and the gryphon. The great scientist of the
thirteenth century, Albertus Magnus, tried to dispel the
legend of the barnacle goose—that it did not breed because
its young were produced from the barnacle tree—saying
that he had seen barnacle geese pairing, laying eggs and
producing young like other geese. But it did not have much
effect. John Gerard, author of one of the great *Herbals*,
swore that he had seen the barnacle tree, and that he had
handled the goslings which hatched from the barnacle.
He wrote this in 1597.

Medicine was about the only field in which the spirit of

active enquiry was not wholly lost. The ancient centre at Salerno maintained a long tradition of medical science; the Greek tradition, preserved in the Arabic writings of Avicenna and Averroes, was studied by Christian scholars in Spain and at Montpellier; and in northern Italy the universities of Ferrara and Padua became famous, both in recovering the old classical tradition and testing it by experiment. Dioscorides, the Greek pharmacologist and contemporary of Galen, had devised a wonderful compound of twenty herbal elements to protect King Mithridates from every form of poison. This recipe was re-discovered, and the botanists tried to identify the plants. Such were the beginnings of a new biological discipline.

This period saw also Ferner, the physician, Paré the first great surgeon, and the Belgian anatomist Andreas Vesalius, whose dissections proved that much of Galen was inaccurate. Dissection of the human body had been disapproved of because of the *luz*, a supposedly imperishable bone at the end of the spinal cord, which was thought to form the nucleus of the resurrection body. Vesalius was suspect because he said he could not find the bone, and left its identification to the theologians. At one time Vesalius shared lodgings with John Caius, the famous doctor and co-founder of the Cambridge college which bears his name. Unlike Vesalius, Caius held Galen to be infallible. Once, when President of the Royal College of Physicians, he ruled that a young man named John Gale, who had been heard to criticise Galen, should never be licensed to the College until he had published a full recantation of his errors.

John Caius was also a friend of the great scholar Conrad Gesner of Zurich, who by the time of his death in 1566 at the age of fifty had written ninety books, ranging from a Greek–Latin dictionary to an enormous four-volume

G

Historia Animalium with illustrations, and a projected history of plants for which he had collected fifteen hundred pictures, one hundred and fifty of which he had painted himself. He was also a keen mountaineer, becoming the patron saint of the Alpine Club. He was a doctor, and died carrying out his practice in the plague.

So we come to the seventeenth century and the birth of the modern world. The first half of the century was taken up with intense struggles, military, political and religious, but after the Commonwealth and the Puritans there was a great burst of exploration. The Pilgrim Fathers sailed abroad, and at home one generation produced Newton in the world of mathematics, Halley in astronomy, Boyle in chemistry (now no longer alchemy), Woodward in geology, Ray in botany, Tyson in anatomy, Mayow in physiology, not to mention such great doctors as Thomas Sydenham and Sir Thomas Browne. Contrasted with severe religious restriction on the Continent, imposed largely by Calvin and Luther, the Church of England, and other religious bodies in Britain, were glad to support this scientific work as being a religious concern for the works of the Lord. So John Ray, the greatest naturalist of the period, could name his last work *The Wisdom of God in the Works of Creation*.

The gulf which separates this ordered world of the late seventeenth century from that of Shakespeare a hundred years before is vividly illustrated by Charles Raven with an episode in the life of John Ray when he went up to Cambridge and persuaded his first friend, John Nidd, to join with him in setting up a cage for frogs where they could observe their habits. In the same year a woman was put to death in Cambridge for keeping a tame frog, on the charge that 'it was her imp' and so an agent of the devil.

Gradually the old folk-lore was critically examined and rejected as unsatisfactory, not least effectively by Sir Thomas Browne of the city of Norwich is his *Pseudodoxia Epidemica*. He bade the medical profession remember that there are two books in which wisdom can be found—the Scriptures, and the book of nature, and that the two are complementary.

Two of his contemporaries at Cambridge, Henry More and Ralph Cudworth, contended against the mechanistic philosophy of Descartes. Cudworth postulated his theory of 'plastic nature' with an innate drive towards creativity and adventure. Ray insisted on an element of design in creation to explain the correspondence between an organism and its functioning, and was interested in the living creature in its environment—how, for instance, does a newborn chick recognise a danger-cry from its mother? The coming development of machinery and industrialism was to provide a very different background for the study of living creatures.

This sudden flowering of genius in Britain ceased as suddenly as it began, around 1720. The years 1700–1850 certainly saw a total transformation of the social scene. At the beginning, society was agricultural; at the end, industrial. The machine, based on the steam-engine, had set the pace. Physics and chemistry wrested the dominance from the biological sciences, and mathematics was the standard of scientific precision. To sketch the progress in science it is hardly possible to do more than give a list of names, and these must be mainly French. In the early eighteenth century stands Réaumur, physician and entomologist. In 1732 was born the Royal Academy of Surgery under the great Jean-Louis Petit. In 1783 Lavoisier, who had identified and named oxygen, finally annihilated the four-element theory first propounded by Empedocles. Buffon, with his *Histoire*

Naturelle cast doubts on the creation of the world in 4004 BC and received a severe reprimand from the Catholic Sorbonne. Lamarck laid the foundations of a theory of evolution. The study of bacteriology made astonishing progress, culminating in the classic victory of Pasteur over rabies and anthrax. Yet Bernard, Pasteur's contemporary, began his first professional lecture with the words, 'The science of medicine, about which I am supposed to lecture, does not yet exist'.

While clinical medicine made such astonishing progress it is perhaps not surprising that the study of mental illness lagged behind: it was a baffling and unattractive field, and those who had the misfortune to be deranged suffered an imprisonment worse than that of criminals. For a hundred and fifty years, since their official persecution ceased, there were no proper hospitals for their care. They were treated like animals, or worse, under charge of ignorant and brutal keepers. The scandalous conditions at the York asylum provoked a public enquiry in 1815, as a result of which it was discovered that the surgeon who had been in charge for ten years was himself insane, was generally drunk, and spent much of his time in a strait-waistcoat: yet he continued to attend his patients. The conditions of the place make sickening reading. Well into the nineteenth century a visit to a lunatic asylum was a common Sunday outing, as enjoyable as a visit to the zoo.

One of the first great steps forward was taken in Paris in 1793 when Philippe Pinel, physician superintendent of the Bicêtre Hospital, unchained his patients. He forbade blood-letting and ducking, two standard treatments, and every form of violence. Such a personal concern for the insane marked the beginnings of modern psychiatry.

At the same time in Paris Anton Mesmer proclaimed his

theory of 'animal magnetism'. His idea of a universal magnetic fluid was nonsense, but his practice of hypnotism which went with it was not. In the nineteenth century, before the discovery of anaesthetics, hypnotism was used for operations, and was developed by the famous neurologist, Charcot, at the Salpetrière Hospital in Paris.

In 1885 a young neurologist from Austria arrived on a travelling fellowship to study under Charcot. He learned all he could about patients under hypnosis, and on returning to Vienna described some cases of hysteria he had seen in men. The President of the Viennese Society of Medicine said this was impossible. A surgeon, refusing the young man access to one of his hysterical patients, asked him if he did not know that 'hysteria' came from 'hysteron' meaning womb; how then could a *man* be hysterical? The student's name was Sigmund Freud.

It is perhaps worth pausing on the threshold of the twentieth century to reflect that the three men who above all have shaped the pattern of its civilisation were German-speaking Jews—Karl Marx, Sigmund Freud and Albert Einstein. All of them rejected religion, and all of them produced a secularised version of the Old Testament vision, Marx substituting the classless society for the New Jerusalem, Freud substituting the 'id' for the indwelling love of God, and Einstein mapping the Creation with his special theory of relativity. Is it possible that through these wayward prophets we may be helped to rediscover the deep purposes of God for his universe?

Karl Marx does not much concern us now. Einstein stands to the twentieth century as Newton does to the seventeenth. Einstein's relativity theory, first published in 1905, together with the quantum theory which Max Planck propounded in 1900, have decisively destroyed the

Newtonian picture of the universe as a box-like space with bits of matter moving around with absolute velocity which are theoretically measurable. The one constant against which absolute velocity could be conceived was the aether, and Clerk Maxwell's theory of electro-magnetic waves cast doubt upon the traditional model of the aether. Einstein's work introduced a new working theory into physics, that physical quantities must be defined by the operations which are used to measure them. Thus all velocities cease to be absolute and become relative to some other body. Furthermore, the length and mass of moving bodies is not constant, as Newton supposed, but they contract according to our measurement of them, and the faster their motion the greater the contraction.

The billiard-ball picture of the universe was finally exploded by the quantum theory which showed that an atom was not at all the simple basic piece of matter the physicists had hoped for. Atoms were broken down to two types of electrons, positive and negative, but their behaviour was very awkward to explain. At times their behaviour demanded an explanation in terms of an electrically charged particle, but at other times in terms of a packet or quantum of waves, similar to light waves. Even light waves would not behave in a proper manner; at times a wave motion was adequate, but at others a shower of particles seemed to be demanded, and so photons appeared on the scene.

Another important side-effect of the quantum theory is the well-known 'uncertainty principle', namely that the act of measuring a very small atomic entity itself disturbs it. We cannot even assume that an electron has anything as definite as a position.

So the way we look at the universe today is different in two important respects: the god-like position of the scientific observer has been abdicated in favour of an admission that the observer cannot finally be separated from what he is observing; and the concepts of mass and matter are both relative to us, and are of a complexity at once mysterious and inconceivable. Heisenberg has warned us, 'We have to remember that what we observe is not nature, but nature exposed to our method of questioning' (76, 946).

Seven years before the publication of the quantum theory, in 1893, Freud and a companion called Breuer published a book called *Studies in Hysteria*, in which they sought to show that physical symptoms of hysteria have their root cause in highly emotional experiences of early life which have been repressed into the unconscious mind and are beyond the reach of conscious memory.

These hurtful incidents are too painful to recall, too challenging to the respectable picture a person has created of himself for the conscious mind to bear, and so they become submerged below consciousness, together with the more primitive drives and impulses which may influence a person's behaviour without his being fully aware of them. Although Freud was not the first to see a connexion between hysterical illness and unconscious mental processes, he did discover that conflicting desires and forbidden or painful emotions in the unconscious mind could shape responses which emerge as symptoms of illness or abnormal attitudes of mind. By way of treatment Freud devised the process of psychoanalysis by which patients were enabled to recall, often over a period of years, emotionally wounding incidents, often connected with sexual experience. When the patient could recognise these for what they were he could be helped to cope with them. This process was often accompanied by an outburst of pent-up anger, resentment, or hate directed against the analyst, but Freud welcomed this as a purgative for the patient's emotions. Freud also found patients loving him and becoming strongly dependent on him, as well as hating him and even attacking him. His partner Breuer had been frightened by these transferences of emotion, and by the wave of unpopularity attending the publication of Freud's findings, and ceased his association with him. But Freud, after many years, learned how to use this transference as a part of the healing process. In his book *The Interpretation of Dreams*, published in 1900, Freud sets forth his belief that dreams are generally the expression of a repressed desire, a sort of code-language or cartoon of the unconscious mind, and if rightly interpreted can give invaluable knowledge of deeply buried desires or fears which often go back to early childhood, even to birth itself.

We cannot now go more deeply into Freudian theory, the ego and the super-ego, the Oedipus complex or the Freudian slip-of-the-tongue; nor can we trace the schools of psychiatry which sprang from Freud, notably that of Adler who saw a craving for power and importance rather than sex as the basic drive; and of Jung, the son of a Swiss clergyman, with his theory of the 'collective unconscious', and his distinction between 'introvert' and 'extrovert'. There are in America today some thirty-two different schools of psychiatry, and any psychological statement is inevitably a matter of controversy. Nevertheless some assessment must be attempted.

Freud had been taught by men who maintained that the only valid principles for understanding the workings of the human body were those that could be derived from physics and chemistry. They rejected any kind of 'vitalism' in biology. Freud, accordingly, set out to construct a 'scientific psychology' using the same theory of causality. He wished to see all mental activity explicable in terms of the interaction of unconscious mental forces; and he thought that if these could be accurately plotted and measured, psychology could be a precise science like physics. In fact, however, the evidence did not allow him to be so deterministic. He refused to predict whether a person would develop a neurosis, and if he did, what sort it would be. He did claim that if a person had a neurosis, a particular event in childhood could be seen to be the cause. This, it has been pointed out by Charles Rycroft (*46*, 14), is more like the work of a historian or linguist than that of a scientist: not the elucidating of causes but the interpretation of their meaning. His most famous work is called *The Interpretation of Dreams*, not *The Cause of Dreams*.

Thus psychoanalysis may be seen as a biological theory of meaning. The analyst, meeting the patient in his consulting room, tries to establish *rapport* with him, but finds the lines of communication blocked. He tries to discover the history of the illness and its origins in infancy, so that this *rapport* may be made more effective, and has as his instrument a long experience of the meaning of the cryptic things which the patient says and does. His task is like that of a linguist meeting a strange tribe and trying to map its language. To enter into the sphere of meaning is, of course, a risky business, but psychiatry does start with at least two presuppositions, that to be aware of some reason for one's mental ailments is better than the wilderness of no-reason, and that the way to more satisfying personal relationships is through a personal relationship, even if it is a very carefully and clinically controlled relationship. It is not sufficient to have a tape-recorder in place of the therapist. There is an assumption here, not always granted by psychiatrists, that the self is 'a psychobiological entity which is always striving for self-realisation and self-fulfilment . . . sharing with the animal and plant world the intrinsic drive to create and re-create its own nature' (*46*, 21).

Freud himself declined to consider the problem of meaning, alleging that living itself provided meaning enough. He dismissed the notion of God as an undesirable external prop resorted to by those who needed an infantile sense of security and protection; but this was his own value-judgment and in no sense a scientific conclusion. It seems likely that the God which Freud rejected was a God of false transcendence, modelled on an obsolete three-decker universe. He never seems to have considered the immanence of the Christian God nor the overwhelming importance which St John attaches to love as the foundation of Christian living. The Christian neglect of the doctrine of the Holy Spirit (who, according to St Paul, communicates the deep things of God to the deep heart of man (1 Cor 2.9–16)) here reaped its full reward. If Marx represents the divine judgment upon the church for its neglect of social righteousness, Freud represents the divine judgment on the church for its neglect of the immanence of the Lord the Spirit.

The tragic events of 1914–1918 accentuated the work of Freud in two ways: the loosening of sexual moral standards found a specious support in his theories; but, more important, the incidence of nervous breakdown, officially labelled 'shell-shock', put psychiatry to the test. At first, those suffering from acute anxiety states were shot; those lucky enough to convert their anxiety into an incapacitating symptom began to be treated for neurosis when it was realised that the human body can take only so much emotional punishment before going on strike. There are many cases, recorded in detail, of soldiers paralysed in legs or arms, blind, deaf, or dumb, where this symptom became part of a solution to an intolerable conflict between a sense of honour and a sense of fear. It was the same mental mechanism which confined Elizabeth Barrett to her bed for twenty years to escape an impossibly tyrannous father, but enabled her, after she had eloped with Robert Browning at the age of forty, to climb Italian mountains the next year, and two years afterwards to bear him a son. Charles Raven tells of a meeting with Professor Muirhead of Birmingham, 'a hard-headed Scottish philosopher', a day after he had visited the great psychiatric hospital at Littlemore outside Oxford where Dr J. A. Hadfield was practising. Muirhead said, 'You ought to have been with me yesterday. I saw miracles; I saw things the like of which you would have to go back to the New Testament to parallel' (*40*, 110).

B. SYNTHESIS

During the last hundred years medical science has made astonishing and spectacular advance. It has found partial or complete cures or preventive measures for most of the great killing infectious diseases—smallpox, typhoid, cholera, diphtheria, meningitis, tuberculosis, pneumonia, and polio-myelitis, and has in the process created vast new problems, such as the economic threat of over-population, difficulties about the prolongation of life in those who can scarcely be called alive, and the rationing of a limited amount of medical care to a far greater quantity of need. It is conceivable that before the end of this century a majority of people in this country may have to exercise a conscious choice about the time of their dying, a matter which will pose some nice problems to the medical profession!

In spite of all this progress, the hospitals of our land are no less full, and indeed if the number of hospital beds were doubled tomorrow patients could be found to fill them. The nature of their ills, however, has changed, and along with this is taking place, often reluctantly, a change in the basic appreciation of illness and the nature of healing. A few years ago the Regius Professor of Medicine at Oxford was asked, 'What is the most significant and promising area of research in medicine today at Oxford?', and he replied without hesitation, 'The relation between body and mind in the cause and cure of disease'.

This approach to human sickness and healing is, of course, not new; but its detailed and accurate clinical investigation is new and is producing results which are of immediate relevance to all who are concerned with the wholeness of man. The term 'psychosomatic', first traced to the year 1818, was introduced into common circulation in America by the researches of Dr Flanders Dunbar about 1935. The word itself is unsatisfactory as it still preserves the old Cartesian duality of mind and body, the ghost in the machine, which the new approach is concerned to break down once for all, and at the present time a replacement has been found for it in 'holistic medicine' or 'whole-man medicine', with the reminder that man's wholeness includes above all things his relationships with other people—and with God.

Such an approach has been forced upon doctors because of the brute fact that a vast number of sick people who are not 'out of their minds' do not have any definite bodily disease to account for their illness. It is reliably estimated that (in the U.S.A.) about a third of the patients with chronic illness who consult a physician fall into this category. About a further third have symptoms which are in part dependent upon emotional factors although organic disease may be present as well.

Nineteenth-century study of disease, as taught for example by Virchow, started with the diseased cell, moved from there to alteration of the physical structure and so to functional disturbance. The twentieth century changed the order in some situations (for example, in some heart disease)—functional disturbance, leading to disease of the cell, leading to structural alteration. There is now a volume of evidence to show that preceding the functional disturbance there has often been psychological disturbance. The extent of these psychogenic influences (a phrase only to be used for lack of a better one) must briefly be considered as they affect every aspect of the body's working.

We may well start with the heart, because this has from ancient times been taken as the seat of the emotions (though not by the Hebrews). The language of poetry and common speech speaks of 'light-hearted', 'broken-hearted', 'hard-hearted', 'chicken-hearted', 'heavy-hearted', 'faint-hearted', and may rightly be taken as a primitive sort of body-language. After all, palpitations as a symptom of anxiety were well known before Freud wrote about them. The whole field of anxiety symptoms connected with the heart is covered by the title of cardiac neurosis. About this doctors are divided. Some recommend as treatment helping the patient to understand how his heart is registering the anxieties of his life-situation. Others maintain that this neurosis is perpetuated by the doctors' own anxiety.

Organic disease of the heart is a much more serious affair, and coronary disease is one of today's principal fatal diseases. Its causes are obscure, and each year brings out a new fashion in aetiology—excess of fat in the diet, too much sugar, or not enough exercise. Twenty or more years ago Dunbar sketched a personality profile of those who suffer from heart disease:

It is characteristic of people who suffer from heart disease that they are hard workers, driving themselves without mercy and apparently enjoying it. . . . They were proud of the long hours they worked, and incidentally resentful of the little appreciation they got for it. They were not in the usual sense, however, victims of overwork. They were victims of the psychological circumstances which were responsible for their apparent ambition. These patients were remarkable in the apparent strength but actual extreme brittleness of their defenses. They were strong only so long as a highly unified, rigidly crystallized life role turned out to be something to which they were culturally well adapted and which they found rewarding. But their brittle shell covered a mental poverty or insecurity which had no other defenses once the shell was cracked. It seemed to make little difference whether the shell was broken from without or within. The result was rapid transition to a bodily ailment (*6*, 126).

This pattern has been questioned by medical researchers, and it lays itself open to all the difficulties of abstracting from so complex a thing as 'personality', but it has recently received striking confirmation from a study carried out at the Mount Zion Hospital, San Francisco. A team selected 3,524 healthy men between the ages of 39 and 59 in 1960. Each was examined for high blood pressure and other symptoms associated with heart disease. The men were also classified according to income, job and emotional make-up. Those with a high competitive personality went into 'type A'; those relatively free from urgency in their jobs and outlook into 'type B'. Since 1960 seventy of the men suffered heart attacks, fifty-four from 'type A' and sixteen from 'type B'. Of the nine who died, eight were from 'type A'. The report says, 'the results clearly indicate that the presence or absence of a particular overt behaviour pattern' was a danger sign for the heart, and the behaviour pattern is of excessive drive, aggressiveness, ambition and preoccupation with competitive activity.

The stomach ulcer is the best-known psychosomatic complaint, and has collected around itself a variety of popular legends, that it is, for example, the affliction of business magnates, amongst whom it may be regarded as a badge of success. In fact, nowadays the incidence is distributed fairly evenly between the sexes, and is by no means confined to the driving, aggressive type with which the coronary is associated.

The most organically-minded doctor cannot deny that strong emotions have a direct physical action upon the stomach. This has been observed and recorded by two American doctors, Wolf and Wolff, who used for their purposes a laboratory assistant called Tom, who because of an accident to his oesophagus, had to feed himself through a direct passage into his stomach. They write (*61*),

A normal condition showed that acid was being continuously secreted in small amounts. In fear or sadness the acid secretion became inhibited, and the mucous membrane of the stomach paled as the blood concentration tended to decrease. When Tom was angry or resentful his stomach flow of acid increased. His mucous membrane flushed as blood concentrated itself and stomach contractions increased in frequency and vigour.

In brief, an ulcer appears to develop thus: emotional disturbance sends an unduly large number of impulses to the stomach by way of the autonomic nervous system (that system over which the owner has no conscious control) perhaps by two different paths. These impulses cause the overproduction of hydrochloric acid which is necessary, in correct proportion, for digestion. Simultaneously tension develops in the muscles of the stomach, which are controlled by the autonomic nervous system, causing strangulation of the blood-vessels supplying the stomach lining. The local areas of anaemia then lose their protective film of mucus and become vulnerable to the hydrochloric acid, and so an ulcer forms, which can be seen by X-ray.

The answer to the question, 'What causes an ulcer?' is, therefore, a complex one. In medical terms the disease must be labelled psychogenic. Neurogenic is not good enough. The nerves do not cause the disease; they only transmit the message. To cut the nerves, as is sometimes done, is, as Dunbar says, like cutting the telegraph wires to avoid hearing bad news. The news will get round sooner or later by other, and perhaps more damaging, paths. To find the underlying cause it is necessary to go beneath the surface, in this case, of the conscious mind. What is generally found is a person whose deepest longing is to depend on someone—mother, husband, wife, friend, but who at the same time is afraid of being a clinging vine and so strives for independence and responsibility, often giving the appearance of a go-getter. He may very well not be at all short of love, but he has so buried this yearning for dependence that he cannot be satisfied by the ordinary run of life; his hunger takes him consciously to ever-increasing independence, and unconsciously (and primitively) to food—which he does not need, and cannot digest. It has been well said, to eat is human; to digest divine.

At the other end of the digestive tract, next to the bowels, is the colon, the seat of a puzzling and difficult disease, ulcerative colitis—an acute inflammation and infection of the lining of the colon. For the Hebrews the bowels were thought of as the seat of the emotions, and not without reason because the digestive tract is the oldest part of us, from the perspective of evolution, and acts as a sounding board for our deepest emotions.

Case histories of colitis patients portray, for the most part, weak personalities, self-centred and strongly dependent particularly on the mother or mother-substitute. They are sexually immature and give up easily. There are frequently emotional conflicts in the background connected with engagement or marriage, and married life tends not to be very successful. The onset of the disease is often connected with an emotional crisis such as the death of a near relative. Some investigators claim that almost anyone could present these characteristics at some time or another, but this is to misunderstand the matter. No claim is being made that these situations are the cause of the disease. Every disease has many 'causes'. There seems little doubt that they play an important part in the whole disease-pattern, and must be taken into account for a complete cure. There are strong similarities in behaviour between a person suffering from colitis and one suffering from depressive illness, and it is possible that these are alternative ways, bodily and mental, of expressing the same conflict.

Tuberculosis has a very long record of recognition as a psychosomatic disease, a description by no means invalidated by the discovery of the tubercle bacillus. The bacillus is everywhere, and most people are infected at some time in their life, but few develop the disease. It seems that invading bacilli are not killed but imprisoned in a guard-room of living cells where they may languish harmlessly until our dying day. If, however, our resistance is lowered, the prisoner breaks out from his guard and trouble starts. Many factors have a part in lowering resistance, and physical ones like malnutrition and bad housing are not the only ones. Towards the end of the last century the great medical teacher, Sir William Osler, warned his profession that the fate of the tubercular depended more on what they had in their heads than on what was in their chests. In 1884 Sir Thomas Allbutt stated in his Goulstonian lectures, 'Perhaps the disease most largely found in neurotic families beyond their neurosis is *phthisis*' (the old name for tuberculosis, the same in meaning as 'consumption')', and thirteen years earlier he had recorded his suspicion that *phthisis* may develop in women after disappointment in love. In 1797 Hufeland had noticed in the background of his patients' lives 'a mournful disposition of the soul', and in 1689 Morton in his *Phthisiologia* observed a 'long and grievous passion of the mind'. Galen, around AD 200, saw the disease springing *hectica ex ira ac maerore*—from a consumptive anger and grief— and as early as 1500 BC Hindu doctors put down grief as one factor in the development of tuberculosis.

These medical hunches have received precise confirmation from the work of David Kissen, who has recorded in his book *Emotional Factors in Pulmonary Tuberculosis* (*18*, *56*) a controlled investigation into the emotional factors preceding the onset of tuberculosis in his patients' lungs. In very many cases he found such factors to be present and the outstanding type is what he calls 'a break in a love link', as, for example, a break or threatened break in a romance, engagement, or marriage. He also found that in patients who subsequently relapsed, emotional factors were more frequently apparent than in those who did not, and in

90 per cent of such patients the type of factor was the break in a love link. He concludes that there is a strong suggestion that deprivation of affection and love plays an important part in the onset and relapse of tuberculosis. These patients appear to be especially in need of love and affection.

George Day, speaking from long experience as superintendent of a tuberculosis sanatorium, records the close connexion between a patient's life-situation and a change for better or worse in his physical condition.

A young man, forced into the family business for which he had no zest or aptitude, slowly went downhill until his father saw the light and allowed him to pursue the vocation he had set his heart upon. I have seen a middle-aged man improve when he became engaged; and then, when he discovered that his young fiancée was sleeping with one of his friends, turn his face to the wall and die within a month. One of my most memorable patients was a young girl who hung fire for *eighteen months*, getting so far and no farther; up four hours a day and walking about four hundred yards. If we tried to increase her activities, she would show unequivocal clinical deterioration and would have to be put back on absolute bed rest for a while, to start all over again. Then her jealously possessive mother, whose senile dementia had for some years been Pauline's constant anxiety, was certified as psychotic and put away in a Mental Hospital—for good. Pauline, who dearly loved her mother, shed some natural tears for a couple of days, and then started to get well; and within two months her three cavities, each larger than a walnut, which to our knowledge had been present for at least eighteen months and had been slowly worsening, completely disappeared. Six weeks later she had reached full graduated exercise and was discharged—back to her typist's stool: part-time for three months, and full-time thereafter.

None of these patients could you call psychiatric cases. The emotions they felt—frustration, grief, anxiety and hopelessness—were perfectly natural in the circumstances. Call them psychosomatic if you like, but for my part I prefer to regard them as suffering from crippling of the spirit: just as Falstaff's spirit was broken by King Henry's brutal renunciation, and never recovered; just as when his Joan is taken from him, Darby has no heart for the business of living (*79*, 202).

A glandular reaction to fear is the secretion of thyroxine by the thyroid gland. The effect of thyroxine is similar to that of adrenalin, but it works more slowly and is designed for longer periods of stress. The disease of hyperthyroidism, or exophthalmic goitre, is the result of over-activity of the thyroid with an excessive production of thyroxine. It is accompanied by a swelling of the thyroid gland in the neck, and a protrusion of the eye-balls—in a set look of terror. Patients who suffer from this disease frequently tell of a period of profound emotional stress shortly before its onset, often of a terrifying quality. Surgical removal of part of the gland helps to control the production of thyroxine, but does not come near the basic cause of the glandular upset.

One of the disorders which has been most responsible for bringing doctors to realise that psychological factors produce physical results is that known as *anorexia nervosa*. The symptoms, normally in young women, are extreme emaciation with lack of appetite, the total stoppage of menstruation, and an appearance of much older years. At root these patients show a profound repudiation of sexuality, and their starvation assists them in this by making them look unattractive. There is also an effect on the pituitary gland which controls the menstrual function, but it is a functional not an organic disorder, because if the condition yields to psychological treatment, the gland resumes its proper purpose. The disorder seems to be a bodily expression of a deep rejection of life, and the treatment calls for the discovery of the cause of this rejection, so that life may again be tasted and enjoyed.

Hippocrates was aware that an attack of asthma could be brought on by some violent emotion, but it is only in the last twenty-five years that detailed study has been done on correlating symptoms with these emotions. Listening to a patient's wheezing will tell a doctor a good deal about the constriction of his bronchial tubes; listening to a patient's life history can tell him much about the constriction of deep and important emotions, and the two are intimately connected, not causally, but in dependence upon each other.

An asthmatic attack can be precipitated by contact with some substance to which the person is allergic (a term coined in 1906). But how and to what degree the patient reacts to this allergen depends on many factors; hereditary, environmental, as well as emotional. From the emotional side an attack is often precipitated by a situation which threatens the person's dependence on his mother or mother-figure, either by physical separation, or by a temptation to which the person is exposed. A boy slept in the same bed as his mother until he was eleven and was always emotionally dependent on her. At twenty-six he married against her wishes, and had his first attack of asthma. Such an attack is in effect a suppressed cry of rage. It may also be a suppressed cry for help and comfort, for the emotional conflict can also be against wanting to re-establish such a dependency. Some asthmatics say they have never cried for years, and sometimes a severe asthmatic attack stops completely if the patient has a good cry.

Asthma is well known in small children (often allied with eczema), and here it has been found that in a very large number of cases the children have been smothered by over-protective parents. Either the children have been very much wanted, or, on the other hand, have not been wanted at all, but the mother, feeling guilty about this, attempts to compensate by over-fussing. The sins of the parents are indeed visited upon the children and, in the case of asthmatics, often until the third and fourth generation.

Skin troubles highlight the problem of causality in disease, and dermatologists are divided in their assessment of what is to blame. One reliable estimate reckons that of 17,000 patients seen in one year 45 per cent had skin conditions in which emotional factors were believed to be important. One of the principal emotions seems to be a repressed hostility and anger either against someone or something in the environment, or a punishing of self for entertaining these hostile feelings, or a certain masochistic satisfaction. The skin is not only an important layer of contact between the inner and outer worlds but seems also to be a sensitive organ of expression.

Many people have several allergies at a time—skin troubles, asthma, some digestive upsets; and Dr Dunbar comments, 'A physician experienced in the psychosomatic aspect of these conditions can often predict with accuracy whether a patient suffering from one of them today will come back with another at the next visit' (6, 202).

The eye has long been recognised as a powerful organ not only of expression but also of receiving impressions. For the Hebrews the eye was an indicator to the whole personality, an 'evil eye' being idiomatic of a mean or ungenerous nature. Making eyes at people has long been recognised as a powerful means of communication. Seeing is a highly complicated process involving both the central and the autonomic nervous systems, and the latter, the unconscious one, is a well-known victim of shock or anxiety. Hysterical blindness became in the First World War a familiar consequence of shell-explosion or gassing but was eventually found to be treatable by psychotherapy. Micklem quotes in detail (*32*, 112–13) the history of an army pioneer aged forty-one who lost his sight in September 1914, was discharged on pension as permanently unfit early in 1915, and was examined every six months afterwards. In November 1918 he was admitted to hospital, the very picture of the blind beggar of the street; unshaven and unkempt. When he was able to open his eyes his pupils were dilated and there was no trace of reaction to light. After two hours of explanation and encouragement he began to see again, and the next morning he could recognise distant objects; that evening he could read large letters at a distance of twenty feet. Four months later he was working as a watchmaker.

Freud recognised that a precipitating cause for blindness may come from within the personality, often through a sense of guilt arising from the sight of a forbidden object. It is, he said, as if an accusing voice addressed the person, 'because you have chosen to use your organ of sight for evil indulgence of the senses, it serves you quite right if you can see nothing at all now'.

There is little doubt now of a direct link between anxiety

and glaucoma. One investigator has discovered in twenty-four out of thirty-six glaucoma attacks a close connexion with specific emotional events. In nine cases the original attack was precipitated by witnessing an accident which resulted in injury or death to someone with whom the patient had intense emotional ties. An ophthalmic specialist has told me of two or three instances of glaucoma he has found in patients admitted to hospital which were not present when he examined them a few weeks previously for another disorder. He judges that the onset here was precipitated by worry concerning the future of their eyesight.

Rheumatism, or to be more precise, rheumatoid arthritis, shows undoubted connexions with its victim's life-situation. I met a woman in hospital terribly crippled in every joint with arthritis, and I asked her if she could connect its onset with any strong emotional shock. She replied that it began on the day in 1941 when she received a telegram that her husband was missing, believed killed, at Singapore; an hour or so later she 'felt her legs go heavy', and the arthritis had progressed steadily ever since.

Miss Olave Hann has done considerable research into problems of stress and personality in the sphere of rheumatology, and she has kindly allowed me to refer to her findings. She writes of the cases under review:

> These are all 'reactions to situations' and it seems doubtful if they are essentially determined, although the ability to tolerate frustration is apparently dependent upon feelings of security and personal adequacy developed in early childhood.
>
> It may be that because of genetic susceptibility and life experience the rheumatoid arthritic was a 'vulnerable child' unable to withstand early thwarting experiences,

with probably inadequate channels of emotional and motor release, especially during the important developmental period 0–5 years. During this period did he develop a low stress resistance with some disturbance of his adreno-cortical balance before hormonal stasis was acquired? It would appear from his inherent factors, infantile experiences, emerged a shy, withdrawn, anxious, inadequate personality in childhood, the prototype of the adult arthritic in this study. Because of inadequate release mechanisms and an inability to 'hit out physically and emotionally', did he become physically and physiologically sensitised towards a certain 'patterning out', an exaggerated psycho-motor tenseness under trauma—a 'stiffening of his joints' to protect himself against his own aggressive feelings?

If in later life he develops certain stress reactions, can we surmise that he has again encountered a life situation which may re-activate a previous 'psychic' patterning?

The overall impression left by the findings is that despite other external contributing situations which often played a major role, personality factors lay at the root of many of their difficulties. . . . In some instances there was a clinging to their problems as the only form of emotional security—unhappy albeit—that they had; they preferred their worries to the emptiness of life without them.

The non-medical observer might be pardoned for supposing that a bone is a bone, and not much susceptible to personality upsets, but this is far from the case. An orthopaedic surgeon has allowed me to use this account of a case of 'Sudeck's atrophy', an unusual complaint, of which he sees one or two instances a year:

Some months after losing her husband she twisted her

right ankle. Her doctor referred her to the Hospital for an X-ray which was reported as showing no bony injury. Her ankle was strapped and she returned home. Two weeks later her doctor wrote saying he was convinced there was a fracture and phoned up the Hospital and another doctor was alleged to have said that there might now be a fracture. The doctor was annoyed about this and the delay in finding another opinion. He obviously transmitted this annoyance and dissatisfaction to the patient who was then seen by me for the first time. I confirmed there had been no bony injury to the foot or ankle though she had some arthritis which had been present for many years. She was treated in plaster but after two or three weeks she developed a terrific grudge against all treatment that was being carried out in view of the fact that she thought 'a fracture had been missed'. I did my best to reassure her, and inevitably and slowly she developed a Sudeck's atrophy and became more and more disgruntled, so I eventually referred her to a colleague of mine at The Royal National Orthopaedic Hospital in London. He confirmed the diagnosis of Sudeck's atrophy and advised a certain line of treatment which was subsequently carried out. Her leg was treated in plaster for twelve months, after which she had prolonged and repeated physiotherapy and she was only discharged five years after the original injury and just able to walk with one stick. The X-rays are very interesting in that they show a progressive rapid decalcification of all of the bones of the left lower extremity.

The surgeon's opinion is that the intense animosity and resentment which the patient showed was a principal factor in the disease—even to the physical disintegration of bones, of which he has X-ray evidence. The standard text-book on orthopaedic surgery makes no mention of psychogenic factors in the matter.

Medical science of the last hundred years has eliminated many fearful scourges. One, however, remains undefeated, despite unprecedented millions of pounds spent in research: cancer. So notable has been the lack of success that some investigators are wondering whether the main line of research is the right one; they suggest that instead of focusing interest on the cancerous cell, they might do better to look at the cancerous person, especially as, it seems, most people over middle age have cancerous cells in their body, although the malignant process remains in check.

Last year a conference of doctors took place in New York devoted to *Psychophysiological Aspects of Cancer*, and from its report (*76*) some striking conclusions emerge from detailed statistical studies into the personalities and life-situations of cancer patients. Each report in itself is open to criticism, but taken together there is a significant area of agreement among them. A study in New York of 450 adult patients with cancer revealed that 72 per cent of them, compared with 10 per cent in a control group, had a childhood and adolescence marked by feelings of isolation, followed by a period in which the individual lived a meaningful life, and finally experienced 'loss of the central relationship and a sense of utter despair, and a condition that life held nothing more for them'. From Scotland came a report showing that men with a poor outlet for emotional discharge appear to have more than four-and-a-half times the cancer rate of those with a moderate outlook—irrespective of whether or not they smoked or how much they smoked. From Rochester, New York, came a report that in a series of over a hundred cases of leukaemia or lymphoma in adults, the condition developed when the patient was harrassed by 'a number of losses or separations' with understandable feelings of sadness, anxiety, anger or hopelessness. An independent report from Liverpool, of the findings in twenty women with cancer of the uterus, described the patients as of 'an anxious disposition combined with an inability to share troubles' which 'had led to a depressed state of mind . . . and an attitude to illness akin almost to personal defeat'.

Two important conclusions seem to emerge from this kind of study. First, a physical chain of causation from emotional shock or strain to carcinoma can be postulated with a fair degree of probability, from the hypothalamus via the pituitary gland, to the endocrine glands, producing an upset in hormonal regulation which may affect, for example, cancer of the breast or prostate in some cases. This is not a simple causal chain, and many factors enter into it.

Second, several authors in this report conclude that most of our 'cause and effect' language is obsolete and misleading. One suggests that 'hopelessness and carcinoma may be evidences from two frames of reference of the same process and therefore not directly related in a causal chain of sequences' (76, 875). Another says, 'To me it seems to be a *meaningless* question to ask whether the physiological process is causing the psychological state, or the psychological state is causing the physiological process. Both are arbitrary descriptions, in arbitrary terms, of a particular global process, and it is for this reason that I think long discussions about what is most important or basic in such a process are irrelevant, misleading, and quixotic' (76, 1053).

Another paper contains this interpretation:

Although to the social evaluative self, tumors may

appear to be disgusting, dangerous, and foreign, on the deepest and most archaic level of primary process fantasy the creation of a tumor may be as important and meaningful to the cancer patient as is the creation of a symphony to the musician or a plastic form to the sculptor (76, 844).

This sketch of the relations between religion and medicine lays no claim either to completeness or to impartiality. Its principal aim is to show that the mechanistic models used to portray the inner working of nature, based on a Cartesian dualism and on the mathematics and physics of the eighteenth and nineteenth centuries, are now admitted to be inadequate in the understanding of much human illness—and this from the side of scientists, many of whom have no religious axe to grind. Man can, of course, be analysed physically and chemically, as he can be biologically and psychologically; but he is, in himself, more than the sum of his parts. Man in his wholeness still remains at heart a mystery, and man's wholeness is now known to be vitally dependent on his relationship with other people, and, Christians would add, with God.

This recovered emphasis on the care or cure of the whole man, that is, man in his social (and religious) setting, is much to be welcomed, and harmonises in some remarkable ways with the Old Testament insight into man's nature.

It may well be that medical science is on the verge of the computer age, when a person's ailments are programmed on to punched tape and fed into an international computer-system which will store in its mechanical memory the accumulated medical experience of centuries, and from this provide a diagnosis. Nor need we regret such a prospect—provided that *all* the relevant information is fed in. It must seriously be considered whether not only pulse-rates and blood-counts are relevant, but also such factors as the patient's ability to give himself in love to other people, to live with himself and an awareness of his own inadequacies, to cope with strong emotions like anxiety, anger, or hopelessness, in the depths of his being. A computer can only give out the results on information which has been fed in, and it must be asked whether satisfactory answers can be given in all cases without categories very like religious ones being given their due weight.

These conclusions do not necessarily shed immediate light on the problem of miracles. We are not claiming that all the illnesses recorded in the Gospels are 'psychosomatic' in the sense that they belong to the group of diseases which are today labelled as psychosomatic; or that the Lord's methods of healing were those of present-day psychotherapy. It does, however, seem reasonable to claim that today the field is much wider open to an appreciation of at least the possibility of miracle in terms of the impact of one uniquely and supremely whole and holy person upon a disintegrated humanity.

6. An Examination of the Healing Miracles in the Four Gospels

How can the healing miracles of the gospels best be approached? We have argued at length that they must not be approached with modern scientific presuppositions only, because the language of science can never do justice to the notion of 'miracle'. Some modern Christian scholars have evaded the difficulty by, to all intents and purposes, scrapping miracles altogether. Bultmann writes (*Kerygma und Mythos* I, 48, quoted 26, 75–6),

> One cannot use electric light and the radio, or in cases of illness call in the aid of modern medical and clinical methods, and at the same time believe in the world of spirits and miracles of the New Testament. And anyone who believes that he himself is capable of doing so must clearly realise that, when he explains this as the attitude of Christian faith, he makes the teachings of Christianity incomprehensible to and impossible for our present day.

And again, even more strongly,

> They are not works of Christ, insofar as we understand by the work of Christ the work of redemption. Consequently, in the discussion the 'miracles of Jesus', insofar as they are events from the past, must be radically exposed to criticism, and it must be argued with the greatest severity that the Christian faith has absolutely

no interest in proving the possibility or reality of the miracles of Jesus as events from the past, and that this could on the contrary merely be an error. If Christ stands before us as the Christ preached to us, then the miracles of Christ can only enter into consideration insofar as they form part of the preaching of Christ, that is to say as testimony.

Miracles, he adds, are not suitable for confirming faith,

for they leave anyone the choice to convert them into a causality which he understands (*Glauben und Verstehen* I, pp. 214–28, quoted *26*, 32–3).

There is no opportunity here to examine in detail the basis of such an attitude, but it seems to indicate an advanced state of theological schizophrenia: reason is divorced from revelation; the present from the past; redemption from creation; preaching from the sacraments; the individual from the community; mind from matter.

Clearly if these assumptions were granted there would be no point in proceeding with any examination of the healing miracles. Nothing reliable could be established about the original events, and even if it could, it would have only marginal relevance to Christian faith.

Bultmann is a leading representative of the school known as Form Critics, who derive their name from their policy of seeking to establish the *kērygma*, or proclamation about Jesus, from a detailed study of the shape or form which the spoken tradition about the words and works of Jesus took amongst the earliest communities of Christians. They have given up the attempt of the Liberal Protestants of the early years of this century to create a Jesus of History who could be entirely separated from the church's interpretation of him; instead they seek to formulate the church's interpretation of him, separating this almost entirely from any certain knowledge of what sort of a person he was and what he did and said. The most that they allow is that we can have some access to what his followers thought he was and did and said, but we have no means of checking whether they were right or wrong, and anyhow this does not matter. So long as the preaching about Christ (or 'the Christ-event') satisfies the needs of twentieth-century man it is enough. But the Form Critics can offer no historical reason (and would not want to) for the emergence of the Christian church out of the events recorded in the gospels. As R. P. C. Hanson pertinently observes:

> It is therefore legitimate to conclude that Form Criticism explains all the phenomena presented by the gospels—except the reason why there should be any phenomena at all (77, 38).

The Form Critics assert that the gospel material has been cshaped by the needs and concerns of life in the early church communities. But most of what we know about these needs and concerns comes itself out of the gospels. So it becomes perilously easy for the argument to be a circular one, and the final judgment purely subjective. When the edited material contains the criterion for editing it is very difficult to know what (if anything) is original and what secondary.

Many writers of this school reject as original, in doctrinaire fashion, anything which resembles features from contemporary religious life in the Greek-speaking (Hellenistic) world, any parallels from Rabbinic sources, though most of these date from a good century after the time of Christ, or anything which might be considered as a fulfilment of Old Testament prophecy. There is considerable divergence

I

among the various writers as to what may be considered original and what developed.

They have also formulated 'laws' governing the ways in which a story was altered in the course of tradition. They maintain that details of time and place are lost as the piece of tradition is worn smooth in the telling. But at the same time they see any small details which might identify time, place, or participants as fictitious embroidery added to give an appearance of truth. Thus if such details are absent this is proof that the narrative is in a secondary state of development, and if they are present, this also is proof of a secondary state of development! 'Heads I win, tails you lose.'

The degree of caprice shown in these procedures is astonishing when judged by any ordinary historical standards. Bultmann, for example, gives pages of parallels to healing miracles of the gospels drawn from contemporary writers. One of those quoted is an account of cures performed by Vespasian at Alexandria, as recorded by the historian Tacitus (*History*, 4, 81). It is worth quoting at length:

One of the common folk of Alexandria, known for his blindness, flung himself down before his [Vespasian's] knees, begging and sighing for a cure for his blindness, on the advice of the god Serapis, . . . and he begged the emperor to deign to moisten his cheeks and his eye-sockets with his spittle; another, with a sick hand, begged the emperor, on the advice of the same god, to tread on him with his foot. At first Vespasian turned away, laughing, but when they persisted he now feared the rumour that a failure would cause, and then was encouraged by their pleas and the voices of the coaxers; finally he commanded that physicians should examine whether such blindness and impotence could be cured by human effort. After lengthy consultations the physicians judged that the power of sight of the one had not been destroyed and would return when the impediments were dislodged, and that the crooked limbs of the other could be restored if beneficial power were applied; this was perhaps after the heart of the gods, and the emperor had been chosen as the divine instrument; finally, if the cure were successful the fame thereof would accrue to the emperor, whereas if it failed, scorn would be the lot of the unfortunate couple. And so Vespasian, with a glad countenance, and believing that all was open to his fortune and nothing more was unbelievable, complied with the urgent prayers, which the crowd standing by watched with rapt attention: at once the hand could be used again and the daylight shone again for the blind man.

Apart from the cure and the mention of spittle, this story might well be used to point the contrast with the miracles of Jesus in the matter of Vespasian's initial contempt, his fear of failure, his being persuaded against his will, his resort to doctors' opinions, and his self-seeking motives. The verdict of Dibelius (*From Tradition to Gospel*, p. 96) that 'by telling such tales, the pre-eminence of the Lord Jesus could be demonstrated and all other rival gods who were worshipped could be driven from the field' is preposterous.

Other Form Critical judgments may be seen clearly in the Pelican Commentary on St Mark's Gospel (*34*) written by D. E. Nineham, and these are referred to below in the treatment of individual miracle stories.

How may these stories best be arranged? A classification by literary 'forms' is possible, for example the 'short story' or the 'pronouncement story', but the Form Critics do not themselves agree about the placing of some incidents. Classification by types of illness is possible (as Loos, *26*, 339–589), but this blurs the distinction between the evangelists and their different aims and methods. Classification by types of treatment has been attempted by Weatherhead (*58*, 49–50)—type 1 being those cures which involve the mechanism of suggestion; type 2 those involving a more complicated technique; and type 3 those involving the support of other people—but this is to prejudge many issues and to use medical categories which many would regard as not proven. The method which seems to present fewest difficulties is to start with those in Mark's gospel, taking them in Mark's order, considering their parallels in Luke and Matthew where they exist; to proceed with those related only by Luke and Matthew either together ('Q') or independently ('L' and 'M'); and to finish with those recorded by John.

1. *The demoniac in the Capernaum synagogue*
   Mk 1.23–28 ‖ Lk 4.33–37

Mark starts his account of Jesus' ministry by stressing the Lord's authority. He has just previously (verse 22) referred to the strange new authority of his teaching; this now is reinforced by a casting-out of a demon or demons (exorcism) in the synagogue on the Sabbath. Mark tells us very little of what Jesus actually taught; he is more concerned to present a challenging portrait of what he did, and thus of what he was. The portrait here is sketched in terms of warfare and victory over demons. The phrase *what have we to do with thee?* in three places in the Old Testament occurs in a context of military interference (e.g. Jdg 11.12). One of the final conquests of the Messiah was to be over the devil (Rev. 20.10), and Mark takes this opportunity of making plain to his readers that this was the nature of Christ's warfare—not against the Romans—as Paul also does to the Christians at Ephesus. 'For we wrestle not against flesh and blood, but against principalities, against powers, against the rulers of the darkness of this world' (Eph 6.12).

The mind of this unfortunate victim was indeed darkened. He was mentally deranged, though it is not easy to identify the type of illness. The opinion of medical writers varies between hysteria and epilepsy or a combination of both. A psychiatrist has suggested to me that it was epileptic psychosis with paranoia, which until recently was mistaken for schizophrenia. The 'tearing' in verse 26, and the 'throwing' in Lk 4.35 point to an epileptic seizure, and the paranoid sense of being persecuted is apparent in the man's hostile reaction to Jesus' approach. The healing is miraculous in its suddenness and completeness, and the onlookers, though familiar with exorcisms, are *amazed* (a strong word in Greek). It is more than just a non-conforming event. It contains a disclosure for which the only adequate language is that about God's activity.

Has modern psychiatry any light to throw on this healing process? Archbishop Anthony Bloom (who is also a qualified doctor) tells of a psychotic person who was so deeply withdrawn that he had not spoken a word for nine months. He sat by his bedside in silence, for four hours, and the patient began to speak. Is this perhaps a faint indication of the power of a holy presence on a deranged mind? Doctors argue about the origin of schizophrenia—is it disturbance in relationships, or chemicals in the brain, or both? But the basis of psychotherapy is the use of 'relatedness' for healing ends. It seems reasonable to suppose that if the relatedness between Jesus and his Father was of a unique kind, this superhuman quality could be used to restore relatedness to a mind at odds with itself.

I know thee who thou art, the Holy One of God. Sometimes there is more sanity in the distraught words of the insane than there is in the calm observations of the sane (See R. D. Laing, *The Divided Self*, chapter 2, p. 19). At all events St Mark uses those words to let his readers into the secret of Jesus' identity at the beginning of his story.

2. *Peter's mother-in-law, and other healings*
   Mk 1.29–34 ‖ Mt 8.14–17 ‖ Lk 4.38–41

This small episode was doubtless preserved because of the personal link with Peter and his family (Matthew and Luke do not mention the presence of James or John).

There is no means of identifying the illness because fever was looked on in the ancient world as a disease in itself rather than as a symptom of various diseases. The remarkable feature is the complete recovery of Peter's mother-in-law who, instead of being weak, as would normally follow a period of fever, at once got up and served a meal. This could have been achieved by hypnosis or even by strong suggestion, but we do not have sufficiently detailed evidence to be sure. The teaching-point of the story would no doubt have lain in her immediate readiness to serve rather than just enjoy a wonderful cure.

3. *The cleansing of a leper*
   Mk 1.40–45 ‖ Mt 8.1–4 ‖ Lk 5.12–14

The setting of this episode varies in the three accounts. For Mark it comes as the climax to a series of healings; in

Matthew it follows Jesus' descent from the mountain; Luke sets it *in one of the cities*, omitting to notice the law forbidding a leper to go inside town walls.

Leprosy was the most dreaded of all diseases, and is the only one for which the Old Testament gives a detailed description and regulations (see Lev 13–14). It was the task of the priest to identify the disease, excommunicate the sufferer, and certify a cure. This was not on hygienic but on ritual grounds, because leprosy was regarded as direct punishment from God for serious sin, and a solemn summons to repentance for the whole community. Of seven cases in the Old Testament four are caused by the direct intervention of God, and three are healed by him.

Does the Biblical term 'leprosy' describe the same illness as 'Hansen's disease' (as leprosy is now technically termed)? There is some doubt about the symptoms as described in Leviticus; and reference is made there to the possibility of cure. There has been no known cure for leprosy before the discovery of sulpha drugs, and leprosy seldom, if ever, cures itself. The answer seems to be that it was the genuine disease, though it may also have included other severe skin complaints, as for example psoriasis. This can be an agonising and defacing disease: its aetiology is obscure, but it is sometimes connected with severe emotional disturbances. Among the signs accompanying the arrival of the Messiah the cleansing of lepers is specially singled out (Mt 11.5 || Lk 7.22).

Mark certainly understands the disease here to be leprosy, and all three accounts contain the fateful words, *Jesus . . . put forth his hand, and touched him*. In so doing Jesus violated the law and put himself outside the pale of the religious community. Instead of *moved with compassion* we should almost certainly follow those manuscripts which read *moved with anger*. Anger at what? At the disruptive forces of disease and sin in the domain of Satan. These are vanquished by a decisive word, *I will*; *be thou clean*.

Jesus had no argument with the religious establishment of Israel, and told the cured man to report to the health authorities for a certificate.

If the disease was leprosy, the cure was wholly outside our knowledge. If, however, it was psoriasis or something like it, then the emotional impact of Jesus' acceptance of the outcast man might very well, within the terms of our experience, have played an important part in his cure. We do not have enough evidence to be certain.

4. *Healing of a paralysed man*
  Mk 2.1–12 ‖ Mt 9.1–8 ‖ Lk 5.17–26

The previous episode showed clearly that Jesus had no quarrel with the religious authorities. The present one shows clearly that they have an important quarrel with him. This story is in fact the first of five 'controversy stories' in which Mark portrays the growing opposition to Jesus from Scribes and Pharisees.

Matthew, as often, shortens Mark's version, but preserves all its main features. Luke shows by his phrase *let him down through the tiling* (verse 19) that he was thinking of a town house with tiled roof, rather than the Palestinian house with a flat roof of clay or turf. The episode is colourful, indeed it was dismissed by Woolston in 1729 as 'monstrously romantick'. There is a certain clumsiness of grammar between verses 10 and 11 in Mark which has led some commentators to exclude the conflict with the Scribes in verses 6–10 from the original. Nineham (*34*, 92) goes so far as to suggest that these verses were invented by the early church to justify its claim to forgive sins by its own experience of working miracles! But the way Jesus poses the challenge in verse 9 is striking and unusual and looks like an original reminiscence.

The story in its present form turns on Jesus' claim to be able to forgive sins. This, as the Scribes know well, is the prerogative of God alone, and not even of his Messiah. But a visible demonstration of forgiveness is not easy. A miracle could be 'laid on' to prove his power, but this is contrary to Jesus' whole manner. It seems certain, therefore, that he saw some connexion between sin and the man's paralysis, though not necessarily the simple link of wrongdoing and punishment.

We are familiar today with 'conversion hysteria' whereby a person confronted with an intolerable situation converts his anxiety into a physical symptom. Wartime stress in a soldier torn between a sense of honour and a sense of fear often produced paralysis of legs or arms which removed him for the time being from an unbearable situation. Young and Meiburg (63, 108) quote the case of a seventeen-year-old boy admitted to hospital

with the chief complaint of loss of feeling in his lower extremities. The only abnormal medical finding was a strained ligament to which the boy had given way completely. This young man was bounced off a tractor while ploughing and landed on his back. The next morning when he attempted to get out of bed he felt numbness in his legs and refused to budge until seen by his local physician who referred him to the hospital for evaluation. He had been warned earlier by an uncle that masturbation would 'eat the marrow out of his backbone', and his mind reacted to his back pain by saying, 'This is it. It finally got me'.

The same authors (*63*, 110) suggest that the earliest clinical case recorded in the English language concerns a conversion reaction. At St Bartholomew's Hospital in twelfth-century London

> there was a young man, Osberne by name, whose right hand was fixed to his left shoulder. His head, pressed down to his hand, lay immovable. It was impossible to move the hand from the shoulder, or the head from the hand. When the man approached the altar of the Blessed Apostle Bartholomew, with lamenting tears, he humbly besought his mercy. And he desired graciously to be heard. When his limbs were free, he and all those who were present with worthy praise magnified God, who is marvellous in his Saints.

5. *The man with a withered hand*
   Mk 3.1–6 ‖ Mt 12.9–14 ‖ Lk 6.6–11

This is the last of Mark's group of five controversy stories. The crux of the matter here is Jesus' observance of the Sabbath. It is generally assumed by those present in the synagogue that Jesus *can* heal; the question is, *will* he? He does, in a public and decisive fashion. Jesus raises the level of controversy to the principle of creativity set against destructivity. There is little evidence in the gospels that Jesus intended to do away with Sabbath observance altogether. Nor is Jesus adjusting the law to suit hard cases; the Pharisees did enough of that. He stands before them as himself the agent of a new creation (as he was the agent of the old), and his warfare against all that hinders the new creation, including sin and sickness, can brook no delay. To allow the kingdom of Satan scope for one unnecessary day is to allow a further day's death and destruction in the world, and this Jesus cannot do. The challenge which he presents is not the choice between a strict or lenient reading of the Law of Moses. It is the challenge of himself, his own person and mission and message. What manner of man is this?

Concerning the nature of the man's illness we cannot be certain. If the withering was the result of, say, poliomyelitis, the healing is outside the terms of our experience. If, however, it was a type of functional paralysis (as illustrated in the preceding section) which had gone uncured for a long time, it would have resulted in some atrophy and shrinking. A cure resulting from the impact of Jesus' personality would in that event be much easier to understand.

6. *Healing of the Gadarene (or Gerasene) demoniac*
   Mk 5.1–20 ‖ Mt 8.28–34 ‖ Lk 8.26–39

This exorcism is related by Mark with unusually full detail. The degree of the victim's insanity, the completeness of his restoration, and the destruction of the swine which accompanied it, must have made an indelible impression on the minds of the disciples who were with Jesus. Matthew abbreviates the story by half, greatly reducing its impact, and records two demoniacs not one. This is perhaps to make up for the healing of Mk 1.21–28 which he has omitted. The scene of the healing is agreed to be near the modern village of Khersa on the east side of the Sea of Galilee. Gadara is six miles from the lake and Gerasa is thirty.

The story is naturally told in the popular idiom of demon-possession, which may account for several of its difficulties for the modern mind. Since this was the recognised cause of madness it is not surprising that the victim understands his own illness in these terms. Jesus addresses a simple word of command to the unclean spirit to come out of him. The madman is sane enough to know that an attempt is being made to cure him, and he resists it strongly—perhaps with an oath *I adjure thee by God* (verse 7) which he had learned from previous unsuccessful attempts at exorcism. Jesus establishes personal contact with the man in the simplest way, by asking him his name. This might have been interpreted as an attempt to gain power over the spirit by knowledge of its name, a well-known feature of exorcisms. The man replies 'Legion', and the explanation is offered that he is by way of being occupied territory with 6,000-odd enemies in control. Weatherhead has an interesting suggestion at this point. If the man was psychotic, this might well have arisen from a childhood experience of shock, and none more likely than the witnessing of an atrocity by an occupying legion. The searing impression left on his mind is 'Legion' and this is he. Weatherhead (*58*, 64) recalls a man in a mental hospital in the First World War who had been tortured by the Germans, and the only word he could utter was the word 'Boche'. The demoniac continues to show strong resistance to attempted cure with a request that the demons be not expelled (St Luke's phrase *into the deep* does not refer to the sea, but to Hades, the abyss, the prison-home of disobedient spirits). Jesus, according to Mark's narrative, gives the spirits permission to enter a herd of swine feeding on a nearby hill, and the swine charge down into the sea and are drowned. Some hours or perhaps days later, local inhabitants come to the scene and find Jesus with the demoniac who is quite restored to sanity.

Such a vivid account of the casting out of devils into something else is not surprising, for it tallies exactly with popular belief that a departing spirit would do some damage on its way out. Philostratus records a demon overturning a statue (*Life of Apollonius*, 4, 20) and Josephus similar treatment to jugs of water (*Antiquities*, 8, 48). If the cure included an 'abreaction', a violent release of strong emotion deeply repressed in the unconscious mind, this could very well have served to start a panic of the swine.

This kind of multi-interpretation is not dishonest, nor is it a seeking for the best of all worlds. It is only claiming that this madman's life-situation was open to various methods of interpretation. He interpreted it in terms of violent self-punishment; his neighbours in terms of demon-possession; Jesus in terms of a decisive conflict between the forces of creation and those of destruction; and we may interpret it in terms of manic-depressive psychosis. Such interpretations may all be true within their limits, because they are derived from different frames of reference. What matters for the miracle was that Jesus' treatment healed the man, and with a sure touch Jesus sends him off to tell others about God's mercy so that his attention may be drawn away from himself. The locals, significantly, were more concerned with the loss of their pigs than with the man's recovery of his sanity.

The scene of the miracle is in Gentile territory (hence the pigs, which were unclean to the Jews), and the early church may well have attached particular importance to this event as foreshadowing the eventual mission of the church to the Gentile world.

7. *Jairus' daughter and the woman with a haemorrhage*
Mk 5.21–43 ‖ Mt 9.18–26 ‖ Lk 8.40–56

This is the only example in Mark (and in the first three gospels) of one healing story being set in the middle of another. It may be a literary device of Mark to indicate the passing of time on the journey, but it is more likely an integral part of the earliest tradition. The whole narrative rings true, and abounds with lifelike detail—the name and social position of Jairus, the age of his daughter, the woman's touching the tassel of Jesus' cloak from behind, the anxiety of the woman because of her uncleanness, the names of the three disciples who go in with Jesus, and the homely instruction at the end to give the girl some food. Matthew abbreviates the combined episode to the barest essentials. Luke follows Mark closely, but omits the disparaging detail, *which had spent all her living on physicians*, understandably if Luke himself was one of the profession. (This phrase does not occur in the best manuscripts of Luke, and is omitted in the New English Bible and the Revised Standard Version.)

The comment, *Jesus, perceiving in himself that the power proceeding from him had gone forth*, suggests that behind the incident lies the authority not only of eye-witnesses but the interpretation of the Lord himself. His authoritative words, *Talitha cumi, Get up, my child* (N.E.B.), are preserved in the original Aramaic, presumably because they seemed so authoritative. To suppose, with Nineham, that the words were preserved as a magical formula which would lose its power if translated into a foreign language (*34*, 162) is a desperate expedient.

The note of authority occurs at the outset, for it was the president of the local synagogue who fell at Jesus' feet—a complete reversal of the attitude of the religious authorities so far recorded. The subsequent healing of the woman also continues the theme of religious controversy because her illness had made her ceremonially unclean and untouchable, and Jesus accepts her touch. At the end, the raising of

Jairus' daughter, if indeed it was a raising from the dead, presents Jesus' authority as outside the normal run of human authority.

The healing of the woman

The woman was suffering from some sort of uterine or vaginal bleeding which made her unclean (see Lev 15.25f.), and so for twelve years she had been excluded from all the religious and much of the social life of her people. The cause of this may have been organic, as, for example, fibroids, or inorganic, a 'functional bleeding'. Of this, Weiss and English write:

> In some women such unpredictability and irregularity and lack of rhythmic control physiologically seems to correspond to some weakness in coping with problems, and the bleeding is an attempted solution. Just as it solves a sexual conflict it may also say, 'You see, I am not well. You must excuse me from the duties of a robust existence' (59, 373).

Whatever the cause, the woman summoned up enough courage to approach Jesus—from behind—and touch the tassel of his cloak. At once she felt cured, and he felt power go out of him. In itself this was not unprecedented in the ancient world. 'Power' was the commonest attribute of divinity, and we have already mentioned (p. 8–9) the Hebrew conception of personality as extending beyond a person to his shadow, footprints, or clothes. It is quite possible that Jesus' unusual sensibility to people's needs made him aware that this woman was, in her own shy way, making a demand upon him. What is unusual is that he is not content to let matters remain at this level which could be interpreted as a merely magical one. He insists on confronting the person face to face, a demand which his disciples dismiss as ludicrous (Mk 5.31). The woman recognised Jesus' requirement and *fearing and trembling, knowing what had been done to her, came and fell down before him, and told him all the truth* (Mk 5.33). If only we had a record of that interview! It must have been quite a long one, especially if her complaint was a functional one, as she now unloaded her fears and guilts and inadequacies upon the Lord. But by this her healing was complete. Her haemorrhage had been healed by a physical encounter; her salvation was effected by a personal encounter of trust, for the words, *thy faith hath made thee whole*, require both elements for their full meaning.

The healing of Jairus' daughter

The same demand for trust in the present power of God's kingdom is made by Jesus to Jairus who brought news of his daughter's death while Jesus had delayed on his way. Jesus turned out of the house a noisy crowd of mourners and then demonstrated that resurrection, which was then regarded as God's final reward to his faithful people, could be an immediate and present reality. But the demonstration must be limited to those who have eyes for the reality of the kingdom of God. As F. W. Robertson commented in a moving sermon (*42*, II, 38):

To behold wonders, certain inner qualifications, a certain state of heart, a certain susceptibility are required. Those who were shut out were rendered incapable by disqualifications. Absence of spiritual susceptibility in the case of those 'who laughed him to scorn'—unbelief in those who came with courteous scepticism, saying,

'Trouble not the Master,' in other words, he is not master of impossibilities—unreality in the professional mourners —the most helpless of all disqualifications. Their whole life was acting: they had caught the tone of condolence and sympathy as a trick. Before minds such as these the wonders of creation may be spread in vain. Grief and joy alike are powerless to break through the crust of artificial semblance which envelops them. Such beings see no miracles. They gaze on all with dead, dim eyes—wrapped in conventionalisms, their life a drama in which they are but actors, modulating their tones and simulating their feelings according to a received standard. How can such be ever witnesses of the supernatural, or enter into the presence of the wonderful?

Two classes alone were admitted. They who, like Peter, James and John, lived the life of courage, moral purity and love, and they who, like the parents, had had the film removed from their eyes by grief. For there is a way which God has of forcing the spiritual upon man's attention. When you shut down the lid upon the coffin of a child, or one as dearly loved, there is an awful want, a horrible sense of insecurity, which sweeps away the glittering mist of time from the edge of the abyss, and you gaze on the phantom wonders of the unseen.

Was Jairus' daughter dead? News is brought to Jesus (Mk 5.35) that she is. Jesus silences the mourners with the words, *the child is not dead, but sleepeth* (Mk 5.39). How did Jesus know? He had not even seen the child. Could it not have been a case of trance or coma? It could have been, but the whole weight of the incident is against it. The sleep of death was a commonplace of the ancient world, but the emphasis of the New Testament is on the awaking from

K

death in resurrection (e.g. Mt 27.52; I Cor 15.51f.; I Thess. 4.13–15). Jesus, by his raising of the girl, proclaims himself to be the resurrection and the life, as he does most explicitly in St John's account of the raising of Lazarus (Jn 11.25).

In any event, the physiological distinction between life and death was not of primary importance in the Hebrew way of looking at man (see p. 13). Indeed the phrase used by Luke, *her spirit came again*, is precisely that used in the Old Testament of the revival of flagging power (e.g. of Samson in Jdg. 15.19). Here, as always, the questions posed by the story are: where did the power come from? and to what end was it being used? This episode comes, in Mark, as the climax to a series of miracles, and such a placing suggests that Mark understood the miracle to be a raising from the dead.

8. *The Syro-Phoenician woman's daughter*
Mk 7.24–30 ∥ Mt 15.21–28

This story bears every mark of genuineness, principally on account of the blank refusal, at first, of Jesus to accede to the woman's request, and the popular term of coarse contempt for Gentiles which he uses in his answer. (Dogs were scavengers rather than household pets in those times—no pampered poodles.)

The reason for his refusal is clear. As a Gentile she is outside the range of his mission which is strictly limited to 'the lost sheep of the house of Israel'. There is no question of lack of faith or unworthy motive: she just happens to be the wrong sort of person. But she will not accept such limits to God's love. She claims no right, but throws herself entirely on his generosity. Such whole-hearted trust, including a sense of humour, in the face of every deterrent, receives its reward, and her sick daughter is healed—at a distance.

The story was no doubt preserved in the church's tradition rather as a foretaste of the eventual mission to the Gentiles than simply as a healing miracle, and also as a powerful lesson in perseverance in prayer. Luther loved to dwell on the details of this story and set this woman 'before troubled and fainting hearts, that they may learn from her how to wring a Yea from God's Nay' (57, 372).

As a work of healing there is not much that can be known about it. There is no indication of the nature of the girl's illness, even whether it was mental or physical. It need not surprise us that one who could heal so wonderfully could do this at a distance, using the love of the woman for her daughter as a 'living conductor', as Trench picturesquely puts it (57, 375). We can only make feeble guesses at the mechanism involved, but perhaps telepathy and extra-sensory perception may offer faint clues about ways of inter-personal communication which are still largely mysterious.

9. The deaf man with a stammer
Mk 7.31–37 (compare Mt 15.29)

It is uncertain whether the deaf man here was also dumb or whether he could produce some vocal sounds. The Greek word is *mogilalos*, a rare though not unknown term in late Greek. It occurs once in the Septuagint to translate 'dumb' in Is 35.5–6, 'Then... the ears of the deaf shall be unstopped ... and the tongue of the dumb sing'. Its literal meaning is 'speaking with difficulty', and this is supported by the conclusion of the miracle in verse 35, *and he spake plain*, as if he had spoken unplainly before.

Deafness and dumbness naturally go together because it is very difficult to speak without a sense of hearing. This man may not have been deaf all his life, and his speech-defect may have grown with the length of his deafness. Deaf-mutism is a recognised hysterical symptom, and was often encountered among shell-shocked soldiers. Many cures by psychotherapy are quoted by Micklem (*32*, 118–120).

The use of touch and spittle is paralleled in pagan heal-ings. It is possible that they should be understood in a personal rather than a medicinal sense. It is noteworthy that our records contain no account of Jesus' use of medicine. Spittle might have been seen as a sort of condensation of breath, and thus a specially intimate means of 'spiritual' com-munication. The use of a foreign word of magic is typical of pagan healing stories, but *Ephphatha*, of course, was not a foreign word when originally spoken, and in any case Mark is careful to provide a translation into the vernacular for his readers. The claim of Dibelius that the sighing or groaning of Jesus (a strong word in Greek) is another magical item is dismissed by Vincent Taylor as 'a love for the bizarre rather than sober exegesis' (*52*, 355). The same may be said of Nineham's verdict, 'The vividness with which the act is described may well suggest that St Mark had seen patients treated in this way by Christian healers . . . and it was per-haps for the guidance of such healers that the details were preserved in the tradition' (*34*, 204).

The motive for Jesus' taking the man aside can only be guessed at, but it need not be more than a desire to escape undue publicity. Is it fanciful to see in the verdict of the crowd, *He hath done all things well* an echo of the creation, when God saw what he had made, and behold, it was very good?

10. *The blind man at Bethsaida*
    Mk 8.22–26

This healing story, like the preceding one, has no parallel

in Matthew or Luke. Perhaps they considered the use of spittle an unworthy means of healing. The two stories are similar in many respects (as might well be expected), but the differences are sufficient to allow each story to stand in its own right.

It is the only account in the gospels of a cure being effected by stages, and the details are realistic, especially if the man was not born blind but had some memory of visual images, including those of trees. There is no means of telling more about the nature of his illness.

Blindness was a common affliction, and there are many records of wonderful cures. An inscription at Epidaurus tells of the blind Alcetas of Halieis who dreamed 'that the deity came to him and opened his eyes with his fingers; then he saw the trees in the temple for the first time. When day dawned he left, healed' (*26*, 420 n.). But to conclude as Nineham does, quoting Branscomb (*34*, 217), that here is proof that this story and the previous one 'were developed, if not originated, in the syncretistic atmosphere of the Hellenistic world' is to go far beyond the evidence.

Mark's purpose in putting the story at this point in his narrative is clear. It heralds the turning-point of Jesus' ministry—Peter's recognition of the Messiah at Caesarea Philippi—and forms an ideal conclusion to the first half of the ministry, which was largely occupied with healing miracles, and a link with the second half, which is to be occupied with the attempt to open people's eyes to the Messiahship of Jesus.

11. *The epileptic boy*
    Mk 9.14–29 ‖ Mt 17.14–21 ‖ Lk 9.37–43

Raphael's picture of *The Transfiguration* portrays in classic terms the contrast between the wonder and the glory of the

Mount of Transfiguration and the descent immediately afterwards to the humdrum level of daily life with its sin and sickness, a contrast which may echo the descent of Moses from Mount Sinai to find and confront a rebellious Israel. It is the only exorcism recorded in this latter half of Mark's gospel, and so Nineham concludes that this cannot be its proper place but that Mark has put it here for no apparent reason. Its connexion with the Transfiguration is attested by the three-fold tradition, and the vividness of the narrative points to first-hand recollection. The disciples are not likely to have forgotten its close proximity to the Transfiguration. There is a measure of duplication in the account, and it is possible to separate two strands of tradition, the first in verses 14–19 with 28–29 in which the main interest is in the lack of prayer on the part of the disciples, and the miracle-story proper in verses 20–27 in which the main interest is lack of faith on the part of the boy's father. The duplication is accounted for as adequately by a two-fold tradition of the same event as by a conflation of two different stories. In any case verses 28 and 29 are generally reckoned to be a later addition reflecting the experience of the early church, and *fasting* is not to be found in the best manuscripts.

The boy's illness is one of the few in the Gospels which can be identified with near certainty. The symptoms which are described in careful detail point to epilepsy. (It is strange that Mark describes the boy's history of fits in more detail than Luke, the medical expert.) There is a hystero-epilepsy which reproduces many of the symptoms of true epilepsy, but the disease remains today largely an enigma. It is caused by—or one of its symptoms is—a cerebral dysrhythmia, an irregularity of electrical impulses in the brain, which may be traced on an electro-encephalogram; its onset may be due to physical damage of the brain, physico-chemical disorders in body fluids, or emotional disturbances, and some patients respond to psychotherapy.

Epilepsy was a particularly dreaded disease in the ancient world and for long enjoyed the title 'the holy disease'. It was widely connected with the moon, whence Matthew's description of the boy as *lunatick* (17.15), and Calvin shared Galen's view that the incidence of the disease was influenced by the waxing and waning of the moon. All sorts of anti-dotes were practised, particularly the exorcist's ring. In the temple of Aesculapius at Epidaurus a man from Argos 'saw in sleep in the temple a vision: he dreamed that the deity stood before him and pressed the ring on his finger against the man's mouth, nostrils and ears, and he was cured' (*26*, 404). The secret of the cure of epilepsy by rings was part of the revelation traditionally brought by Joseph of Arimathea to Britain.

Jesus' approach to the sick boy is notably non-magical. There are no charms or incantations, but a calm and careful inquiry into the history of the case, which continues while the boy is experiencing a fit. Then a single word of command to the *dumb and deaf spirit*, and the boy was healed, once and for all.

This is remarkable enough (as remarkable as the fact that Mark records no astonishment on the part of the bystanders, though Luke does—*And they were all amazed at the mighty power of God*), but the main weight of the story lies elsewhere, with the question of faith or its absence. The scribes had no doubt been denigrating Jesus in front of his disciples, and they could not even reply with a miracle. The boy's father appeals directly to the Lord who answers with a prophetic condemnation of a faithless generation. Jesus' reply to the half-trusting father is sharp, '*If thou canst! All things are possible to him that believeth!* (Mk 9.23 RV), and he appears to ignore the impassioned answer.

Faith here cannot be a pre-condition for Jesus' healing: it was out of the question for the boy because he was unconscious; and it was imperfect both in the father and in the disciples, though in different ways. The father doubted Jesus' ability to heal his son, and the miracle for him became a sign of the power and love of God active in Christ, so that he might come to full belief. The disciples had already come to a full belief, but their faith was so half-hearted that it was as yet an imperfect channel for the healing power of God.

12. *Bartimaeus the blind beggar*
Mk 10.46–52 ‖ Mt 20.29–34 ‖ Lk 18.35–43

From the medical point of view, no more can be said about this healing than about that of the blind man at Bethsaida. Only a thorough clinical investigation could establish the cause of blindness, and that is not available. The form of Jesus' command in Mk 10.49 and his '*What wilt thou that I should do unto thee?*' points to the need for a decisive act on the part of the sick man. The vivid detail in verse 50 *casting away his garment* is evidence of the thoroughness of his decision, because a beggar's cloak, being at once bed, overcoat and money-receptacle, was his most important piece of property. If his blindness was functional rather than organic, such an act of faith could well have played an important part in a cure. But this is to speculate.

Matthew records *two blind men* (Mt 20.30) in place of Bartimaeus, possibly because he omitted Mark's previous blind man (Mk 8.22–26), or because he intended to generalise the event.

The name *Bartimaeus* calls forth one of Nineham's most curious pieces of speculation (*34*, 285). Since his laws of oral tradition rule out proper names he recommends the view 'that this story referred originally to a nameless blind man who later came to be identified with Bartimaeus of Jericho, a figure well known in the early church as one who had *followed Jesus on the way*'. Nineham is, however, presumably unable to adduce any supporting evidence that there ever was a well-known figure in the early church called Bartimaeus, or that he came from Jericho, or indeed that any early Christians were connected with Jericho. If a hypothesis needs so much fiction to support it, it cannot support much weight itself.

The theological purpose of the story is clear. More eyes need to be opened than the blind man's. The disciples, just before, in their jostling for the front seats in the kingdom have demonstrated their blindness to its real nature; and the crowd who in a little while are to hail him as a Davidic king, are equally in the dark. This is the first time in Mark's narrative that Jesus publicly accepts the title *Son of David*.

It is possible that the phrase *followed Jesus in the way* may carry overtones of Christian discipleship since *the way* was a common description in the earliest times of Christianity (see Acts, 9.2; 19.9,23; etc.).

13. *The centurion's servant*
Mt 8.5–13 ‖ Lk 7.1–10

This is the only healing miracle related by Matthew and Luke but not by Mark. Verses 11 and 12 in Matthew are found in a different context in Luke (13.29 and 28).

As to the parallelism of this story with that of the nobleman's son in Jn 4.46–54 the scholars are divided, Bultmann, Barrett, Loos and Weatherhead claiming that it is a variant version, and Augustine, Trench, Plummer, Temple and Dodd seeing it as a different event.

A centurion was a senior non-commissioned officer or warrant-officer, roughly equivalent to a sergeant-major. This one was clearly a Gentile, and presumably a regular soldier of the Roman Army. He was equally clearly well disposed to the Jews and their religion (or perhaps their morality), having built them a synagogue (Lk 7.5). He recognises that it is not right for a Jew to enter a Gentile's house, but he goes further in his recognition of Jesus' authority which does not require his coming to the sick man. The centurion's remark about authority is two-edged: as he exercises authority, so does Jesus, which is why he believes that Jesus can heal from a distance; and by the words *I also am a man under authority*, he acknowledges that Jesus' authority itself is derived. It is this insight into Jesus' divine authority which calls forth such high praise, *I have not found so great faith, no, not in Israel* (Mt 8.10).

The medical details of the sick man are not clear. Matthew describes him as lying paralysed and in great pain, Luke as at the point of death. Various guesses have been made about the nature of the illness, as different as tetanus, rheumatic fever, or hysterical paralysis, but they remain simply guesses. It would appear from the narrative that Jesus did not make close enquiries into the nature of his illness, and so there can be no parallel with normal medical practice. The strangeness of the cure is accentuated by its performance at a distance, but if in his person Jesus bridged the gulf between time and eternity, his ability to overcome the limitations of space cannot be ruled out.

14. *Two blind men*
    Mt 9.27–31

This passage, unique to Matthew, does not follow his Marcan source. Some details are similar to the Jericho episode (see pp. 136f.), but all healing-stories necessarily have a good deal in common. It is not necessary to suppose that Matthew has created this episode by 'editing' his later story. It is more probable that he has selected a free-floating item from the oral tradition as typical of the Lord by whom, in the last days, 'the eyes of the blind shall be opened, and the ears of the deaf unstopped', as foretold by Isaiah (35.5).

Jesus does not here publicly accept the title Son of David, but calls the men aside into a house. Faith here is equated with belief in Jesus' ability to heal. The word in verse 30 *straitly charged* is an unusual one, meaning an expression of strongly felt emotion, often of anger; it was used by Mark (1.43) in the healing of the leper.

Medically, nothing more can be said.

15. *The dumb (and blind) demoniac*
    Mt 9.32–35 ‖ Lk 11.14–18.
    Compare Mt 12.22–32 and Mk 3.22–30

The textual situation is complicated. The important part is the controversy about Beelzebub which is related by Mark unattached to a particular work of healing. In 9.32 Matthew connects it with a *dumb man possessed with a devil*, in 12.22 to *one possessed with a devil, blind, and dumb*, with an elaboration of the controversy. It is not impossible that the same argument occurred twice in different settings and was remembered with corresponding variations.

From the medical side little can be said. The man's illness is credited to demon-possession, so there may have been a recognised element of mental instability involved. Hysterical blindness and dumbness cannot be ruled out.

The main interest is, however, theological. The Pharisees

do not doubt Jesus' miracles, but they ascribe them to the power of Satan. (The origin of the name Beelzebub is unknown; there are at least six different scholarly conjectures.) Jesus is happy to acknowledge that healing miracles done by Pharisees derive from the same spiritual source as his own, but, in conjunction with his own person, they are a sign of the arrival of the Kingdom of God and of the overthrow of Satan's rule. If the Pharisees cannot tell the difference between the two kingdoms, then there is no hope for them.

16. *Widow of Nain's son*
Lk 7.11–17

The fact that this story of the revival of a dead man occurs only in Luke does not mean that it is only a quarter as well attested as if it had occurred in all four gospels.

It is true that the story has echoes of Elijah and the widow of Zarephath, with the same words *he delivered him to his mother* (I Kgs 17.23), but these words are what might be expected in such a situation. It is also true that Nain, if it is the modern village of Nein, is not far from Shunem, where Elisha raised a widow's son (II Kgs 4.8–37).

It is also true that there are contemporary claims for raisings of the dead. Apollonius of Tyana is credited with one by Philostratus (IV, 45) in a story which bears several likenesses:

> Apollonius also wrought this miracle at Rome: a marriageable maiden had died, to all appearance, and her betrothed was following her bier, lamenting their uncompleted nuptials, as is the custom, and all the city was mourning with him, for the girl was of consular family. Apollonius, happening upon this mournful sight,

said: Set down the bier, and I will put an end to your tears for the maiden! He asked at the same time what her name was, and many supposed that he intended to deliver the customary funeral oration in order to increase their grief; but by merely touching the body, and murmuring a few words over her, he woke the girl from her coming death, and she found her voice at once, and returned to her father's house, like Alcestis when called back to life by Hercules. The family offered him one hundred and fifty thousand denarii, but he told them that he presented it to the maiden as her dowry. Now whether he had discerned in her a spark of life which had been hidden from the physicians (for Zeus is said to have sent a shower of rain which was streaming from her upturned face) or whether he actually called back and rekindled her departed spirit, is hard to decide, not only for me, but for those who were present at the time.

In view of the fact, however, that Philostratus was writing well over a century after the time of Luke's gospel, if there has been borrowing it is by Philostratus from the gospel and not the other way round. The apocryphal gospels contain numerous raisings credited to various apostles, but these are historically worthless. There are Jewish claims for raisings by Rabbis, but none earlier than the third century AD.

The evidence for the raising of the dead stands in all four gospels (taking Jairus' daughter to be one such), and seems to have been universally accepted in the early Church, as for example by Justin (*Apology*, i, 22, 48), Origen (*Contra Celsum*, ii, 48), and Quadratus (quoted in Eusebius, *Hist. Eccl.*, IV, 3, 2), at a time when there was still opportunity to check with eye-witnesses. And it would have been easier to check in Nain than in Rome.

The internal evidence is persuasive. The name *Nain* survives, though otherwise unknown (but the Form Critics would allot no value to this); the detail of the only son of a widow is preserved; the Lord stops the procession with a gesture, and raises the dead man with a single decisive command; and the effect on the crowd is not an unrestrained joy but fear.

It is a modern Western approach to differentiate sharply between the raising of the dead and, say, the healing of a leper. Sickness for a Hebrew was a form of death in the midst of life, and as far as miracles are concerned there are no degrees of 'difficulty'. Today the dividing line between life and death is becoming less and less clear, with remarkable records of resuscitation from a state which would until very recently have been described as undoubted death: as, for example, the case of a boy of five who was drowned, submerged in the water of a partly-frozen Norwegian river for at least twenty-two minutes when the temperature was −10°C., and then successfully resuscitated by modern medical skill (*67*, 8).

There can be no final 'proof' in the matter of this miracle-story. As with all such stories the reader must decide on a balance of probabilities. It is always open to argue for a coincidental recovery from a death-like trance, but an unprejudiced mind will see as many reasonable difficulties in that sort of explanation as in St Luke's.

Luke sets the story at this point in his gospel to be a fulfilment of the Messianic age pictured in Is 35 and 61, but the interesting thing is that the raising of the dead does not actually occur as part of the Old Testament detail. It cannot be claimed that Luke has devised this story of resurrection to fit the prophecy. It is simpler to accept that he put it here because it was 'one of those things which are most surely believed among us, even as they delivered them unto us, which from the beginning were eye-witnesses, and ministers of the word' (Lk 1.1–2).

17. *The bowed woman*
  Lk 13.10–17

The main emphasis of this story is not the healing miracle as such but the fact that it was performed by Jesus in a synagogue on the Sabbath. The incident follows a serious warning to Israel of an imminent crisis and the challenge which it presented. Will the fig tree bear fruit or will it be cut down? Can they read the signs of the times?

Jesus reclaims for the Sabbath its proper nature, as a day of joyful liberation, freedom from toil, freedom from evil, freedom for God, a veritable foretaste of the kingdom of heaven. Jesus does not defend his breach of the Sabbath; he claims that his freeing the woman so long bound by Satan is the due fulfilment of the purpose of the Sabbath—*ought not this woman . . . be loosed . . . ?* (verse 16).

The Rabbis issued a variety of interpretations of what constituted work on the Sabbath: the stricter is illustrated in one of the Dead Sea scrolls: 'No man shall help an animal in its delivery on the Sabbath day. And if it falls into a pit or ditch, he shall not raise it on the Sabbath' (*Damascus Document* xiii, 22–23). Jesus is not concerned for the nicely calculated less or more, but for an absolute conquest of evil, a present triumph for the power of the kingdom. Such a radical reinterpretation of the Sabbath was only possible for him who was its original framer.

The nature of the woman's illness cannot be assessed with accuracy. Luke gives the detail of *eighteen years* as its duration, and the phrase *a spirit of infirmity* might indicate a mental element in the illness, rather than a purely organic defect. Most of the medical commentators suggest some sort of psychogenic paralysis, and schizophrenia is often accompanied by just such a postural defect often lasting for many years. Even if this was the woman's trouble, her sudden cure with a word from Jesus and the laying-on of his hands remains no less a miracle.

18. *The man with dropsy*
    Lk 14.1–6

This incident theologically is similar to the previous one, though set in the house of a Pharisee instead of in a synagogue. Jesus refers here to the more lenient interpretation of the law about work, in contrast to the stricter rule of the Dead Sea ascetics (quoted in the previous section).

Medically, little can be said because 'dropsy' is not a disease but a symptom of many illnesses, for example of the heart, liver or kidneys. The legs usually, and sometimes the abdomen, become waterlogged owing to failure of the excretory system.

19. *Cleansing of the ten lepers*
    Lk 17.11–19

This is the fourth healing miracle to be recorded only by Luke, to be accounted for, no doubt, by his special interest in the outcast.

Bultmann dismisses the incident as a secondary Hellenistic development of the healing of a leper in Mk 1.40–45, (*26*, 495), despite the fact that Luke has already given his version of this incident in 5.12–14, and despite the fact that in almost every detail the stories differ except the mention of leprosy. Concerning the details of leprosy the reader is referred to the discussion under Mk 1.40–45 (pp. 118f).

Under the scourge of this disease some Jews had forgotten their national distinctiveness so far as to admit a Samaritan to their company. They call trustingly to Jesus (since they may not approach him), and are healed as they leave him, on their way to the Temple authorities for a certificate of health. One alone returns, an outcast of outcasts, to give thanks to God at Jesus' feet, and the clear meaning of Jesus' words in verse 19 is that wholeness is more than physical healing; it includes a grateful awareness of God's special activity in Jesus Christ.

20. *The healing of Malchus' ear*
   Lk 22.50–51 (cf. Mk 14.47: Mt 26.51–52: Jn 18.10–11)

Whereas all four evangelists refer to the cutting off of an ear of the high priest's servant (identified by John as Malchus), only Luke tells of its miraculous healing, though it must be admitted that its manner of performance is far from clear. From the phrase *he touched his ear and healed him* it would seem that the ear was hurt, but not cut off. A variant tradition recorded that the ear was cut off, and Luke has probably conflated the two, with a strange result. Dodd has examined in detail the complex literary tradition lying behind this episode which points to considerable variation in the oral tradition (5, 79).

21. *The nobleman's son*
   Jn 4.46–54

This is the first of John's healing miracles. Before considering it in detail one has to ask, Can it even be put alongside the healing stories of the Synoptic gospels and subjected to the same sort of examination? Does not the very

name 'synoptic' ('seen from similar points of view') rule out
the Johannine tradition as requiring quite different treatment? Ever since Clement christened John's 'a spiritual
gospel' there has been a tendency to suppose that therefore
it is less reliable historically than the others. The nineteenth-
century critics reinforced this view, with the Synoptics
providing 'hard facts' and John 'nothing but abstract
theology in symbolic guise' (to borrow Dodd's phrase;
5, 5). The last thirty years, however, have seen an acknowledg-
ment that there is a good deal of solid theology amongst the
brute facts of the Synoptics, and conversely a good deal of
solid historical tradition amongst the theology of John. The
full case for this contention has been argued by Dodd, who
concludes that 'behind the Fourth Gospel lies an ancient
tradition independent of the other Gospels, and meriting
serious consideration as a contribution to our knowledge of
the historical facts concerning Jesus Christ' (5, 423).

Many commentators have jumped at superficial similarities between John's story of the nobleman's son and that of
the centurion's servant in Q (No. 13), and supposed that
these are variants of the same incident—with John's being
the less reliable of the two. But the differences are considerable. John gives Cana as the place of encounter, 'Q'
Capernaum; John gives a nobleman and his son, Luke a
centurion and his servant; John portrays a man of weak
faith who felt the necessity for Jesus to come to his child,
'Q' describes a man of such strong faith that a mere word of
command would suffice. As Dodd amply demonstrates (5,
189), the shape of the story is much nearer that of the Syro-
Phœnician woman than of the centurion's servant.

John's typical phrase *signs and wonders* appears in verse 48,
terms not viewed with favour by the Synoptic writers.
'Sign' is an important concept in the Old Testament, being

either a direct act of God (Exod 4.8), or a symbolic action, as when Ezekiel drew a picture of Jerusalem under siege (Ezek 4.3); it may be, as in these instances, a sign to Israel—often of warning or judgment—or it may be for the Gentiles (Isaiah 66.19). The word 'sign' was avoided by the Synoptists, appearing only in a pejorative context, though the miracles are for them thoroughly sign-bearing. John's choice of the word was probably governed by its additional use both by stoic philosophers and also in popular Greek religion.

John's difference is one of terminology rather than of essential meaning. Miracles in the Fourth Gospel deepen people's faith—as they do in the other gospels—and as in them they are useless to the sceptical (Jn 12.37–41). Some faith on the part of the father followed Jesus' promise of healing, *the man believed the word that Jesus had spoken unto him* . . ., but John stresses that much more was necessary, and was eventually forthcoming, *so the father knew . . . and himself believed, and his whole house.*

Dodd concludes, and it seems a fair conclusion, that the ideas present in this Johannine passage lie well within the traditional circle and do not need to be accounted for by Johannine theology. 'There is every probability that we have here an independent formation within the common oral tradition' which 'may represent a strain of development later than the principal strains of Synoptic tradition' (*5*, 195).

From the medical point of view the story sheds no more light on healing than do the similar stories of healing at a distance recorded by the Synoptists and discussed above.

22. *The cripple of Bethesda*
    Jn 5.1–9 (18)

The story of this healing in verses 1–9 is similar in shape and content to many Synoptic miracles. The phrase *take up thy bed and walk* is identical with the phrase in Mk 2.9 concerning the paralysed man, and the charge of blasphemy is the same in both, though reached by different ways. Unlike the Synoptists, John's story is prefaced with careful details of time and place, though we do not know which feast is referred to. The name of the pool appears in different forms in the manuscripts—Bethesda, Bethzatha, Belzatha, or Bethsaida—but its locality has recently been established by archaeologists who have found a double pool in the north-east of the city whose remains indicate four colonnades, one round each side, and a fifth dividing the pool in half. The pool would have been reduced to ruins by the Romans in AD 70, and so either this detail of place was incorporated into the tradition before John received it, or else he was familiar with the site and was particularly interested in topography. Careful attention to place-names is a feature of his gospel. The thirty-eight years' duration of the man's illness seems to be a genuine detail; at least it is hard to read any symbolic value into it.

The challenging question, *Wilt thou be made whole?* is in line with Jesus' approach to sick people in the Synoptic records. The leper (Mk 1.40) and the father of the epileptic boy (Mk 9.22) both raise some query about the will or power of Jesus to heal, and in each case the subsequent narrative leaves no doubt that both will and power are present. The further question of the patient's will to be healed is not explicitly raised, though it is implicit in such commands as '*Arise . . . and walk*', and '*Stretch forth thine hand*'. The will to health is implied in the word 'faith'.

If our contention is true that a good deal of illness is an escape-mechanism enabling a person to retreat before un-bearable circumstances into a refuge providing attention and sympathy, then the question *Wilt thou be made whole?*

goes to the heart of the matter. We have no information about this man's illness (it may have been hard to diagnose!), but it is possible that he found a greater reward in being ill than in being well, and, deep down, may not have been so much grieved that someone else was able to reach the curative waters sooner than he. Such a running away from life is a sin, being a denial of the original purposes of the Creator. It is not sufficient in this case for the symptom only to be removed; if it is, it will be replaced by another, perhaps with mental illness instead of physical illness. Is this the meaning of Jesus' severe warning, *Behold, thou art made whole: sin no more, lest a worse thing come unto thee*—? If a demon is cast out a new occupant must be found for the clean and garnished house, lest seven other worse spirits enter into the man (Mt 12.43–45). Jesus finds the man in the temple. The sick man's cure lay indeed in religion, yet religion can itself be an escape from life. After this further meeting with Jesus he *told the Jews that it was Jesus, which had made him whole.* Jesus is the religious answer, but he is never an escape from life.

The narrative slips imperceptibly into discourse, as is the way of the Fourth Gospel, with the weak link in verse 9 *and on the same day was the sabbath*—itself an indication that the story was taken over by John as a unit of tradition. The gist of the argument about sabbath-breaking is contained in the striking words of verse 17 (N.E.B.) *My Father has never yet ceased his work, and I am working too.* As the Son of God, Jesus does what God does. The Jews rightly assess this as a claim to be equal with God, but John has only made explicit here what is implicit in the Synoptics, that Jesus' power to forgive sins is God's power (Mk. 2.7), and that Jesus' power to reshape the sabbath is God's power which shaped it in the beginning (Lk 13.16). The life which Jesus offers is not only life abundant but also life eternal.

23. *The man born blind*
Jn 9.1–7 (41)

Although the incident of the healing of the man born blind occupies only the first seven verses of this chapter, the chapter must be taken as a whole because it is a supreme example of John's creation of a dramatic dialogue growing out of a simple event. It contains the mature fruit of profound and extended meditation on the nature of the person of Christ, here crystallised in the saying, *I am the light of the world* (9.5), that Light which was in the world, and the world knew him not; who came into his own, and his own received him not.

The story of the healing itself is straightforward and similar to Synoptic narrative. The question about the cause of the man's blindness in verses 2–5 seems to be a Johannine insertion, as witness the typical phrase, *work the works of him that sent me*, and the contrasting terms *day* and *night*, although its theology is identical with the passage about the tower of Siloam (Lk 13.1–5): that sickness or disaster is not a punishment for sin but rather the raw material out of which a special decision may be made for or against the kingdom of God.

There seems every likelihood that the name *Siloam* (verse 7, cf. Is 8.6) was contained in the original tradition, though John gives the name an ingenious twist in the direction of him who was sent from the Father and is himself a spring of living water.

Spittle is again used in the act of healing though here mixed with earth to make a 'mud-pack'. A parallel is often quoted from an ancient inscription,

To Valerius Aper, a blind soldier, the god [probably Aesculapius] revealed that he should go and take the blood of a white cock, together with honey, and rub them into an eye salve and anoint his eyes three days. And he received his sight, and came and gave thanks publicly to the god (*1*, 293).

We should perhaps regard the use of spittle by Jesus as not so much medicinal as a kind of breath or spirit materialised, and mixed here into a salve to make its effect longer lasting. The prescription offered to Valerius Aper is a potent mixture of medicine and magic.

Concerning the nature of the cure nothing can be said from the medical angle. It is as absolute a miracle as the next, the raising of Lazarus. The 'difficulty' of the miracle is not as great as the opening of the eyes of the Pharisees whose blindness was incurable because they thought they could see.

24. *The raising of Lazarus*
Jn 11

Around the tomb of Lazarus the critics are massed in battle array. From Renan's claim that the episode is a pious deceit fabricated by Martha and Mary to support Jesus, every shade of scepticism may be found.

The meaning of the chapter, that is to say John's intention, is abundantly clear. Jesus is not only the light of the world, he is the resurrection and the life (verse 25). Into this last miracle story John has poured his full and final understanding of the person of Christ. Faith in Jesus removes the sting of death for all believers; the grave loses its victory once and for all. Martha's confession of faith, *Yea, Lord: I believe that thou art the Christ, the Son of God, which should come into the world* (verse 27), is the heart of the Christian creed, but few readers would suppose that Martha reached this formula of belief during the Lord's lifetime.

It is, in fact, impossible here to extricate primary tradition from John's treatment of it. The whole chapter is composed with a masterly skill which defies any scissors-and-paste treatment. Yet in many ways the whole story bears some striking similarities to Synoptic tradition, notably in the Marcan story of Jairus' daughter. In both there is a delay as a result of which the sick person dies. In both Jesus describes the person as sleeping—though John is careful to point out that he was talking of the sleep of death. In both the sight of the conventional mourning moves Jesus to strong emotion; in Jn 11.33 the word for groaned (*enebrimēsato*) is an unusual one occurring only here and in Mk 1.43, Mk 14.5, and Mt 9.30. There is good reason to believe that this episode has behind it as sound a tradition as lies behind the similar Synoptic narratives. John has taken it and shaped it to his purpose, but this is no more than must be said for the other evangelists.

That the Synoptic gospels do not mention the raising of Lazarus is, like all arguments from silence, a dangerous one, especially when used to deny the historicity of the miracle. Mark's information reflects mainly a northern or Galilean tradition, while John's has a much heavier weighting towards a southern or Judean one. For John, the raising of Lazarus represents the final act which brings to a head the opposition of the Pharisees: for Mark it is Jesus' cleansing of the temple. But the Marcan links of cause and effect are not reliable, and the location of the cleansing of the temple in the ministry is a notoriously difficult problem. As John himself points out (20.30), his book contains only a small proportion of all the signs which Jesus did in the presence of his disciples, and the same must be said for the other gospels also.

The theory has been advanced that the raising of Lazarus is the parable of Dives and Lazarus (Lk 16.19–31) turned into a miracle. The sting of the parable certainly lies in its tail, 'If they hear not Moses and the prophets, neither will they be persuaded, though one rose from the dead', but Dodd has shown (5, 229) that it is the occurrence of the name in the parable which needs explanation, rather than its occurrence in the miracle-story. No parable in the Synoptic gospels contains a proper name, but miracle stories in Mark give us both Jairus and Bartimaeus. It is much more likely that if a story about the raising of Lazarus was circulating in early tradition, the name was absorbed from the event into a parable which took as its core a popular, anonymous folk-tale. It is one thing to draw meaning out of an event (or even to put meaning into it), but it is quite another to invent an episode to give false incarnation to an idea.

For John the raising of Lazarus is the last and supreme sign. It is an 'absolute' miracle, underlined by Martha's crude words, *Lord, by this time he stinketh*. Popular belief was that the soul hovered near the body for three days hoping for a re-uniting, but after four days there was no hope. Lazarus' body *had lain in the grave four days already* (verse 17). It may even be that John intends a miracle within a miracle, in the manner in which the body, bound with grave-clothes, comes out of the tomb before Jesus gives the command, *Loose him, and let him go*. But the degree of miracle is of little concern to John. A life of perfect obedience to the Father will produce wonderful results, and the prayer which Jesus offers (verses 41–42) is not that this work may be done, but that those who witness it may know that it comes from a life lived at every moment in perfect accordance with the Father's will.

The full significance of the raising of Lazarus could not be realised until Jesus had himself been raised from the dead (it is noteworthy that the New Testament almost always speaks thus, rather than of his rising from the dead), but the two events are not logically comparable. Lazarus had to die —again. Jesus' resurrection was to eternal life with the Father from whom he had come. The resurrection of Jesus does not fall to be considered among his healing miracles. Logically it is parallel only to the incarnation: as the incarnation is the basis of all the miracles done by Jesus in his lifetime, so the resurrection is the basis of all his miracles done since.

7. Miracles Then and Now

THE purpose of our journey has not been to prove miracles either ancient or modern. Indeed, it has been our main contention that there is no possibility of being able to prove miracles. One cannot prove a joke: one can only see it and laugh, or fail to see it and not laugh. As seeing a joke proves one's sense of humour, so seeing a miracle proves one's faith in God. Christians must finally abandon the evidentialist use of miracles: it will not work. But this is not to say that miracles must be abandoned, least of all the healing miracles. At a time when some medical men are concerning themselves again with the question of the 'whole man', how he works, and how he fails to work, and how he may be restored to working order, the gospel miracles offer powerful clues as to where this very wholeness may be found.

Science, or the method of investigation belonging to the natural sciences, cannot prove or disprove miracles or the possibility of miracles. All it can do is to say, Here is something outside our experience. It should be quite happy to do this because it is by just such admissions that science advances. A miracle should be a stimulus to science to check the accuracy of its observations, and if the observed results do not fit into the accepted picture, to look again at the picture to see if it should be expanded or altered so that the new data can be fitted in.

Any recorded miraculous event, ancient or modern, is already a matter of history, and must lay itself open to the critical inspection of the trained historian. It is interesting that a new approach to the vexed problem of the historicity of the gospels is being attempted through the comparative study of ancient history (77, 83–90); and professional historians who are not theologians are prepared to give the gospels much higher marks for historical reliability than the Christian demythologisers. Even so, no historian investigates or writes without his own assumptions. There is no such thing as unbiased history, and history as a scientific discipline can never prove miracles. There is always the possibility of error, intentional or unintentional, in the human factor. It seems that the German school of Form Criticism has attempted to escape the question of historical reliability because, smarting from the failure of the Liberal Protestants to delineate a foolproof 'Jesus of History', they cannot bear the possibility of being proved wrong again about the historical Jesus. But such misunderstanding, and the re-interpretation which must follow from its discovery, is one of the inevitabilities of the incarnation.

The strict historical method, in looking at the miracle stories of the gospels, will not fail to see them in their wider setting, which includes their consistency with the teaching of Jesus, with the whole tenor and direction of his life, with the impact which they made upon his enemies and upon his friends, and with the total consequence of his life, death, and resurrection as crystallised in the early church.

It is precisely because miracles are a burning-point for faith that they have encountered so much opposition, which is as much emotional as it is rational. It is a great relief today that from the side of science, particularly in the discipline of medicine, there is a growing recognition that the traditional concepts of physics and chemistry are inadequate and inappropriate to account fully for such a complex process as the healing of a sick person. This, of course, does not prove miracles, but it does stop scientific rationalists from laying down a law that miracles are impossible. We hope we have by now established the point that such a dictum is nonsense.

Little has been said so far about recent occurrences of miraculous healing, and this is a field of investigation to be approached with trepidation. Newspapers love to make sensational headlines out of remarkable cures; services of faith-healing can be relied upon to produce some cripples who throw away their crutches and walk freely for a while; doctors produce the rejoinder, almost as a conditioned reflex, 'It must have been a wrong diagnosis in the first place'; and medical text-books, confronted with hard facts, label them with some embarrassment 'spontaneous cures'. Under such a smokescreen of muddled thinking the British Medical Association declared in its report on divine healing, 'We can find no evidence that there is any type of illness cured by "spiritual healing" alone which could not have been cured by medical treatment' (69). It would have been astonishing if they could.

One remarkable recovery has lain within my own experience which was described to me as miraculous both by the doctor involved and by the patient, though for different reasons. I quote parts of her story (with permission) because it illustrates well the two sides of miracle contained in our initial definition, both *dynamis*, a non-conforming event, and *sēmeion*, a sign of God's especial care. Some would not admit it as a miracle because it was not permanent. In fact, the person had a relapse and died a year or so after the events here described. She faced her death with faith and tranquillity.

The patient, a woman in her middle forties, entered hospital for suspected cancer. An operation revealed severe cancer of the womb with extensive secondary growths. She insisted on knowing the full particulars and so the surgeon told her, and in answer to her question he measured her life in weeks rather than months. After three weeks in hospital she went to convalesce for a fortnight, and then went home. Two weeks later she felt much better, and a further examination by the same surgeon revealed no sign of the expected spread of the disease, and he was able to reassure her that now there was no cause for anxiety. She wrote to me,

> For the whole of my time at T. convalescing, up till a fortnight after coming home . . . I had no hope of anything like complete recovery. All I was hopeful of at that time was that I could be preserved. Mr B. had only promised me that the drugs he would give me could help to keep me fit a little longer.
>
> It may be that I was resting and contemplating but I know that up till that time I have never prayed to be restored, merely to be given strength to persevere. I remember about this time reading about the healing of the leper in Mark 1 and suddenly feeling differently and beginning to pray 'Lord, if it be thy will', and from that time I have been better. . . .
>
> I think the miracle, to me, has been not my healing but the fact that I was able to face up to the knowledge of my condition.
>
> I think I told you on one occasion that I would not have described myself as particularly devout. I have always had a simple faith but I would not have said that my trust in God was equal to an occasion such as this.
>
> Here I will quote from a scribbling I did in hospital, and perhaps you will glean something from this.

I felt no sense of shock (referring to the surgeon's breaking the news)—I had expected it—but a feeling of sadness because I know I shall leave great sorrow behind me. People were already praying for me and I am convinced that the power of their prayer supported me then. I could feel it, and continue to do so. I remember thinking: This is what is meant by 'Underneath are the everlasting arms'.

Later I wrote,

Lest I appear self-satisfied I admit that the two or three weeks before I came here were a very anxious time indeed. I had moments of terror when I went about praying rebelliously, beseechingly, childishly, 'Please, God, don't take my life away', and my nerves were ragged with lack of sleep and worry. . . .

However when I was told, after investigation, that my case was in a secondary stage with extensive spread, I felt no terror or fear, only gravity and sorrow. Almost immediately I felt a sense of support and being uplifted. . . .

During the next few days my worry completely disappeared and I felt a sense of great peace and happiness. I began to review my life and it ran before my eyes like a film taken in sunshine. . . .

The certainty that God watches us on the road through life, led me to believe that he had decided for me, that the rushing and tearing, the constant race against time, was over, and gradually with hours spent in contemplation, usually in the still of the early morning, I came to this state of peace.

You will see now perhaps why I am convinced that in that lay the miraculous part of it all and that everything else was secondary.

I discussed these events with the surgeon at some length, and he confessed to being quite unable to account for her improvement in terms of medical science. He was sure it was not due to the drugs he gave her. He did concede that in his judgment an important factor in her recovery was the spiritual courage with which she faced the knowledge of her condition.

After I had finished writing this chapter the surgeon looked up the medical details of this patient, and sent me a long communication about the case. The following points seemed to him to be of particular relevance:

1. I had seen this patient on two occasions in the previous year in a state of considerable anxiety and worry, thinking that she had some form of malignant disease owing to a strong family history of this condition. On both these occasions, in spite of careful examination, I was unable to find any evidence of disease at all.

2. Slightly less than three months after the latter of these visits she saw me again with obvious signs of malignant disease in the abdomen: I suspected a malignant ovarian cyst. At operation we found extensive malignant spread within the abdominal cavity, but were unable to find the source of the primary growth; it did not appear to have arisen from the womb or the ovaries and may well have come from the stomach. In view of the extensive secondary spread any operative treatment was quite impossible, and indeed there did not seem much point in submitting her to further investigations to find out where the primary growth had come from, because there was absolutely nothing that we could do about it.

3. In such an apparently hopeless case we thought it worth while trying her on one of the new cytotoxic

drugs which have been shown to have a very useful effect against cancer of some types. At that time we had had little experience of the use of this particular drug. Whether it was the result of knowing exactly how she stood in relation to her life and problems, the result of her own guts in facing up to these problems, or the result of the spiritual assistance which you were able to give her, or indeed the drug itself, remains uncertain; I would think a combination of all of them. I now know from more extended experience of this drug that it was no miracle that her symptoms improved so remarkably during the following few months. It may be helpful for you to know that I think that the future treatment of malignant disease probably lies along these lines, and in fact I have had two cases since then which were just as bad as or indeed possibly worse than the one we were talking about, who have survived over two years from the commencement of treatment and as far as I can see at the moment are a complete cure.

What I want to say is that I do not think that her apparent improvement was the result of any miracle, because this has been repeated as a result of drug treatment in my later experience; but I still think that the remarkable improvement in her whole mental attitude was a miracle, helped perhaps by myself as well as by you and her faith.

The surgeon added that he was by no means sure that these further details would help me with my thesis. The reader may judge for himself. At least his letter shows clearly just how difficult it is to analyse the varied elements in the process of the recovery of a sick person, and how difficult it is, as a result, to be sure of a miraculous element on the

M

physical side. Of the miraculous element on the mental or spiritual side in this instance there remains little doubt.

Any discussion of modern healing miracles must include some assessment of the claims made by the Roman Catholic church for Lourdes. There can be no doubt that some remarkable cures have taken place among its thousands of sick pilgrims. The number of those officially claimed is, however, remarkably small. The figure which Dunbar gives (*6*, 103) of two hundred out of a total of sixty-eight million pilgrims (a figure which has attained a wide circulation, as Weatherhead quotes a Hunterian Orator using it, *58*, 157) must be wrong. She quotes Dr Leuret, the resident physician, as estimating the number of pilgrims at a million a year, but it is probable that this estimate referred to the total number of pilgrims who had ever been to Lourdes. In fact in 1948 15,800 sick pilgrims passed through Lourdes, a figure given by Leuret himself in his book *Les Guérisons Miraculeuses Modernes* (p. 113), and of this total, eighty-three dossiers of cures were submitted to the Bureau of Medical Authentication. Of these, fifteen were retained for further scrutiny, and only nine survived into the next round, that is to say, 0.06 per cent or about one in 1,660 (*op. cit.*, p. 194). Not all of these qualified as miracles. Between 1938 and 1948 only twelve cases were finally placed in the category of 'extra-medical' cures, and of these, four were pronounced by the ecclesiastical committee to be miraculous. In the hundred years since Bernadette Soubirous had her visions, that is between 1858 and 1958, only fifty-four miracles have been claimed, and none were claimed between 1913 and 1946 (*33*, 301 n.). The overall total is remarkably small.

The careful efforts made by the Roman Catholic authorities to discern miracles by scientific criteria are commendable, but are in the end self-defeating. Clearly they rule out flights of fantasy and imagination as well as doubtful products of oral tradition, and there is no reasonable doubt that wonderful cures have occurred. But when their spokesmen claim, as does Monden (*33*, 285), that science not only indicates a constant correlation between the facts of healing and a relevant religious context, but also shows 'that this relation is exclusive: thanks to an exhaustive study it can exclude every other explanation or even every other prospective explanation, and thus prove that the lively connexion with the religious context remains the only constant actually demonstrable which is capable of leading to an explanation of the facts', they are making impossible claims for science, and, be it said also, for the Roman Catholic church, since religion here is more or less identified with that body. The heart of our argument in Chapter 3 has been that science, as such, cannot deal with the concept of miracle at all. It can leave the door open to alternative ways of accounting for non-conforming events, but it can never, by its own discipline, say that religion is the only possible alternative explanation.

In fact exclusive claims of this sort have now been demolished from within the structure of the natural sciences themselves, not least in the modern appreciation of psychogenic factors in sickness and healing. Many of the cures which were labelled 'miraculous' fifty or even twenty years ago, can now be seen in a different light. It is noteworthy that the Roman Catholic authorities sternly disallow from consideration any disease which might be called psychosomatic (Monden still talks of organic medicine and psychology working on different scientific levels, *33*, 287), but many of the cures at Lourdes which he describes are of tuberculosis and cancer. It is now certain that emotional factors can play an important part in the course of both of these diseases. It is true that care is taken at Lourdes to diminish the wrong sort of mass emotion, but a visit there as a pilgrim remains none the less a powerful emotional experience.

The Roman Catholics do themselves a disservice with their undue stress upon the *dynamis* of Lourdes at the expense of its *sēmeion*, especially when they rely upon the physical sciences to substantiate their claims. After all, a pilgrimage is a journey undertaken to deepen faith, and there is ample testimony of new courage and hope and freedom found by many thousands at Lourdes. One physician, who has had cures among his patients, has said,

> Whatever may be said as to the value of bringing to Lourdes each year these hundreds of sick on the chance that one or two of them may be cured, the important thing to me is that all of them are in some way changed, and go back with a different attitude toward their illness and able to help others, whether it be only the fretful patient in the next bed in the hospital to which they return to die, or whether they get well and go out into the community (*6*, 101).

Salvation is more than health, and most of us have had experience of people crippled in body (and sometimes even in mind) who radiate a vitality and a spiritual richness which makes the fittest of us seem only half alive. The worship of physical health is as dangerous an idolatry as any.

Consideration of modern miraculous healing in the light of the Christian tradition raises the basic question of the transposition of the gospel into modern terms, not so much a matter of demythologising as remythologising. What are the invariable factors which must be carried over unchanged, and what the variable ones which we should expect to change? This question leads straight to the heart of the modern theological battlefield, and any engagement is likely to be with wounds, but the issue must not be shirked.

First, then, the invariables. All healing comes from God. It is a dynamic aspect of his kingdom because it is rooted in his nature which is love. He has built into the entire created order a tendency or striving towards wholeness, to which vision Teilhard de Chardin has given powerful expression in his writings. The medievals recognised a *vis medicatrix naturae* and knew that, though a doctor might treat, it was nature that healed. The task of medicine is to annihilate or render harmless invaders which threaten man's wholeness, be they bacilli or viruses, chemical or genetic deficiencies, neuroses or psychoses. So in a broad sense all true medical practice and research is by way of being a religious occupation, however uncomfortable many of its practitioners may feel in this classification.

The miracles of the Bible are particular displays of God's love (rather than of his power) and the love of God is an invariable, though the ways in which it is expressed are infinite in variety. The miracles of Christ do not originate in himself but in the Father. The Synoptic gospels portray them as signs of the near approach of the kingdom of God; St John as a foretaste of the new quality of life, eternal life, which is a present possession for the believer. The early Christians may have healed 'in the name of Jesus' (Acts 3.6; 4.10), but gifts of healing and of the working of miracles were, for St Paul, different gifts of the one Spirit of God (I Cor 12)—the same Spirit by which Jesus had cast out demons (Mt 12.28).

While it is true that St Paul recognised individuals as possessing a gift of healing ability, these are set firmly within the corporate life of the church. The church has been described as the extension of the incarnation, but this definition runs the risk of failing to give due weight to the variable factors involved in the transposition. There is a kind of *imitatio Christi* which is a wooden and unimaginative attempt to reproduce the life of Christ. This must fail because it ignores the vitality of the Spirit within the Christian community. The early Christians made many mistakes in working out the pattern of their common life and doctrine (notably the initial exclusion of Gentiles) which were put right only with great effort, and it took time to adjust to new life in the Spirit. The task of adjustment is not yet finished, nor ever will be.

At least we are rediscovering the vital importance of the community and the quality of its spiritual life and personal relationships. The *alter ego* of the ascended Christ is not the Spirit in the church but the church in the Spirit, and it is a humbling reflexion that much of what it means to be a healing community the church has had to re-learn from modern psychiatric practice.

Perhaps the item of greatest variability is the belief in demons and the practice of exorcism. The Lord accepted this belief and practised his healing ministry within that frame of reference. But the frame of reference has all but disappeared in the modern world, at least as far as medicine goes. Or is it that, having been shown out of the front door by the white-coated clinician, the demons are entering by the back door in the guise of anxiety and the despair of meaninglessness, racial and colour conflict, over-population, and the squandering of the earth's natural resources? Are these the demons which the church of the twenty-first century will be called to cast out? Here, perhaps, is an answer to the old question, Why does St John fail to give any account of the casting out of demons in his gospel, whereas it is such an obvious feature of the Synoptics? He recognised the demonology of his day to be a variable, and to some extent deceptive, frame of reference, and since the aim of his gospel was to be as universal as possible, this was one element which he deliberately excluded. 'Verily, verily, I say unto you, he that believeth on me, the works that I do shall he do also; and greater works than these shall he do; because I go unto the Father' (Jn 14.12).

One principal task which must always be a concern for Christians in the broad field of healing is to keep it fully human, and in view of the depersonalising tendencies at work on all sides, success in this mission will be in the nature of a miracle. Christians have no quarrel with humanism except to maintain that by itself it cannot be itself. If man's highest privilege is to have been made in the image of God, and to have been re-made when that image was defaced, then they cannot attain their full stature on the purely human level. Modern medical science has demonstrated, if demonstration were necessary, how important personal relationships are in the matter of sickness and healing. Christians will welcome this and go further, claiming that a person's relationship with God is the basic fact of his being, a new dimension which in no way belittles other dimensions of being, but on the contrary vitally penetrates them at every point. Divine love and human love cannot be separated into watertight compartments, as St John insists in his First Epistle.

Quite practical results follow. Christians should be concerned that much hospital care, while taking immense pains over a patient's body-chemistry, frequently ignores the patient's visitors, even if a dominating parent leaves a child (often a grown-up child) weeping with humiliation and fuming inwardly with anger and resentment. They should be aware of the harmful tendency of the old-style mental hospital to institutionalise their patients, especially their more capable patients, so that the hospital laundry could be manned and the hospital grounds gardened more easily and cheaply. Christians will continue to call in question the vast prescribing of tranquillising drugs. Above all, Christians will encourage an openness in facing and discussing doubts and difficulties in every aspect of health service, for this is what Christians mean by speaking the truth in love. They will insist that treating symptoms only, while covering up underlying unpleasantnesses, is not doing justice to a patient as a person. They will strive for a greater openness to the realisation of the consequences of serious illness and of death, as with the late Godfrey Mowat, the blind healer, who would not let his friends pray for the restoration of his sight because he had accepted his blindness and found that it gave him an exceptional faculty of seeing into the hearts of those with whom he talked (*60*, *91*).

Such openness meets with fierce resistance, as is apparent from the exciting story told by Dr Denis Martin in *Adventure in Psychiatry* (*28*) of the process of turning a traditional mental hospital, with its repressive régime and authoritarian hierarchy of doctors and nurses, into a community where the personal relationships themselves between staff and patients become a principal item of therapy.

From his experience Dr Martin is in a position to assess the church's achievement as a healing community, not least because many of the patients who came to his hospital were church members. He writes:

Thought of in religious terms, the method adopted in the therapeutic community is that of the redemption of

evil by love. Patients are actively encouraged to share
what they feel to be bad or sinful with the community
and there find acceptance and understanding of it. The
community is encouraged to share the suffering of the
individual through an increasing acceptance of him.
Hostile and rejecting responses are made the subject of
discussion which often reveals them to be defensive
measures because of similar tendencies in the other
members of the community. On the whole Church life is
far too respectable for such a redemptive process to
proceed since for many Christians today religion is a
matter of morality rather than love. But at the centre of
the teaching of Jesus is a cross which is the symbol of
redemption by creative love prepared to suffer the full
impact of evil. The Church needs to recognise this afresh,
not as a controversial doctrine of atonement, but as a
practical way of life, and it seems probable that this will
involve the risk of the surrender of superficial respecta-
bility and conventional morality (*28*, 185).

It needs, perhaps, to be stressed that an accepting community is not the same as a permissive community, if by that
is meant a community which has no standards of judgment.
To be a part of a therapeutic community is a testing experience, and Dr Martin's patients found little peace in his
hospital, but they did find a deep security. Some of them
preferred peace, not being prepared to go deep enough for
the security, and discharged themselves. As St John records
of those who were looking for the security of the kingdom of
God, 'From that time many of his disciples went back, and
walked no more with him' (Jn 6.66).

This is the kind of sphere in which the world may see
God's redemptive work in action. It is not labelled 'reli-

gious', and it is a mistake to suppose that spiritual healing must be non-medical healing. Spiritual healing has been well defined by Dr Lambourne as 'an action done by the love of God through the love of men and women because of their love of God'. It makes no difference whether the act itself is changing dirty bed linen or injecting with penicillin, or listening to a suicidal person for two hours, or praying in intercession, or anointing with oil, or helping a woman to accept life with an alcoholic husband. 'It is the fact that the power of love is recognised as coming from God and being offered back to God through service to the sick man that constitutes it as spiritual healing.' He adds, 'The miraculous thing is that such obedient acts of love offered to God bring new love to the fellow workers, which, fed again into the work can transform it just as a change in ward morale can change the recovery rate of patients with fractures' (*68*, 19).

Healing miracles, then, start with the love of God and operate through the faithful response of his people in every sort of trouble, sorrow, need, and sickness. They are displays of the particular care and concern of God, and are bound to be non-conforming events because obedience to God is never merely natural. They are also divine signs, pointers to the present reality of the kingdom of his love.

8. Personal View from a Hospital

THERE can be few Christians who, having had some experience of hospitals, have not asked themselves, 'Why does God allow this suffering?' Many have gone on to wonder why, if he can still do miracles, there is not some wonderful wand that could be waved to remove such a mass of misery. Some ask themselves whether prayer is not such a means. If they pray with faith and hope for someone they love, why should this not guarantee a miracle of healing? Does God not want the sick person to get better? Or is it a measure of weakness of faith on the part of one who prays?

The reader, if he has persevered as far as this, will not expect quick and easy answers to these questions which are by their nature deep and complex and also highly charged emotionally.

The orthodox Christian view of sickness is that it is a result of sin. But we must be quite clear what is meant by 'sin'. The opposite of sin, as Kierkegaard insists, is not virtue but faith (*17*, 213). Sins may be a manifestation of sin, but only on a superficial level may sickness be ascribed directly to the result of sins, if by that is meant, evil actions. If a man drinks a bottle of gin a day he need not be surprised if he develops cirrhosis of the liver. But when the Book of Common Prayer in the 'Order for the Visitation of the Sick' describes sickness as God's visitation it means a good deal more than this. That service is designed to bring a person's sickness into the context of God's particular and personal dealings; dealings which are specifically likened to those of a loving father for his sons—even if today we are not so happy about the chastening element which is emphasized there.

A deeper understanding of sick people, however, has revealed what is for me, at least, a strange new connexion between sin and sickness. In this country nearly fifty thousand people a year attempt, more or less seriously, to end their own lives. It is normal for a general hospital to admit two hundred such patients in twelve months. Here, indeed, are symptoms of a 'sickness unto death' arising from a despair which is the opposite of faith. Although the Church of England no longer holds suicide to be a sin, it is, in Kierkegaard's sense, one of the most striking symptoms of sin, and one which is without doubt a growing feature of our modern civilisation (*50*, 11–21).

If our contention, argued in Chapter 5 (B), is valid that much of sickness is the body's despairing retreat from intolerable strains of life, often at a deeply unconscious level, may we not see here an out-working of original sin? This much-misunderstood phrase does not refer to a single historical event in the remote past (for the story of Adam and Eve is psychological in significance, not historical, being the story of Everyman in the depths of his being). The doctrine is an attempt to formulate an insight into the distortion which inevitably befalls human nature when it is turned in upon itself. If a person fails to love God he will not be able fully to love his neighbour, nor, for that matter, himself either. An excess of human love can be as harmful as a lack of it.

A middle-aged woman suddenly lost her husband to whom she was devoted, and with whom her whole life was wrapped up. Within a matter of days a virulent cancer broke out in her body. She became intensely depressed, and made more than one attempt on her own life. She was sure that life now held nothing for her. Was the cancer obeying in her body the dictates of her will to die?

A young woman suddenly lost a father and, soon after, a sister of whom she was very fond. She was left at the mercy of a possessive mother and dominating aunt. She developed ulcerative colitis, together with a deep depression, and was operated on for the removal of part of the colon. The operation was successful, but she died a few days later. Had she lost all will to recovery? Had the recuperative power of her body gone on strike?

Few sights have I found more pathetic than that of a young woman, newly married, who was dying of asthma. She had been rejected by her mother as a baby, and had been brought up by a couple whose family history was a chronicle of drunkenness, violence and cruelty. Her medical treatment had been almost entirely concentrated on the condition of her lungs—as if the cure for a weeping woman were to excise her tear-ducts.

Even sadder, perhaps, was the baby born to a mother in her later life who was not only not wanted but was positively resented, and was made to know it. From birth he was covered with agonising eczema, and soon developed asthma as well. He became a 'problem child'.

These are some of the kinds of situations to which the word 'sin' correctly points. The Bible affirms that sin is a corporate thing, with the sins of the parents being visited upon the children unto the third and fourth generation. If there is lacking a lively love of God, the lack will make itself known and felt in all human relationships; and if there is present a lively love of God, this can provide stability and buoyancy in very difficult human situations.

The healing treatment which Christians can provide is love (*agapē*), which is simple enough to say but not so simple to practise. It requires knowledge, because no treatment is effective without some diagnosis. Basically it consists of compassion, an imaginative entry into the sick person's situation, to be with him there and go through it with him. Listening is more important than speaking, and accepting more than judging (which does not mean to say that no judgment is made, or that important things are not said). It might be claimed that this is no more than superficial psychotherapy. Christians need not worry if psychiatry has systematised 'love' into certain techniques. They can gladly learn from them and contribute insights of their own. But in any healing encounter of this kind the quality of the personal relationship is of primary importance. A psychiatrist can only do his job if the patient tells him the truth about the things which matter. Sometimes the patient does not.

The exercise of this kind of Christian love can have quite dramatic results even at the physical level. A young man was in hospital awaiting an operation for the removal of a bleeding peptic ulcer. For half an hour he poured out to the chaplain a story of his own unfaithfulness to a wife who, he said, was lazy and careless. Their marriage had been a shot-gun affair, and they had tried to counter its strains by having more children. The wife was worn out and unwell. Both husband and wife had themselves been illegitimate children, and had known no stability at home. Less than a week after his talk with the chaplain this patient was discharged without operation and with no visible signs of ulcer on the X-ray photograph. The chaplain cannot 'prove' that this conversation was a vital part of the treatment, but he has seen too many similar instances to believe that they are all mere coincidences.

What then of the question of praying for sick people in these kinds of circumstances? If their sickness is a body-language it serves to give warning of deeper trouble underlying. For God to remove the symptom miraculously might be positively harmful, as harmful as removing the pain of a toothache which gives warning of an abscess beneath the tooth. To pray for these people means setting them and their problems in the divine dimension. This may simply mean sitting with them for an hour. It will often mean listening to them (in absolute confidence), for there are few aspects of Christian ministry which reproduce the care and concern of God so accurately. There will be little need to talk about the love of God when it is being practised so energetically and (often) so exhaustingly. Prayer for them will entail intercession, holding them and their needs before God when we are away from them, and it may be connected with such sacramental acts as the laying-on of hands, anointing with oil, and the giving of Holy Communion.

In short, prayer for the sick is neither a substitute for penicillin nor is it a bludgeoning of God to do what he is otherwise unwilling to do. It is rather an enlarging and deepening of the spiritual–personal realm, a conscious offer of room for the Holy Spirit to move and work in. How he moves and works will often surprise us; but move and work he will.

The results of prayer will never be stereotyped, any more than the results of marriage will ever be stereotyped. The most we can pray for is that John or Mary Smith should get better. In a Christian context 'getting better' means becoming a better servant of God's kingdom. We may believe that normally God requires his servants to be healthy (if only because so much of Jesus Christ's ministry was spent in healing sick people). But some of his notable servants have suffered from gastric ulcers, and some of his saints have had distinctly neurotic traits. Bernadette Soubirous, the saint of Lourdes, died of cancer at the age of thirty-five.

The Christian approach to suffering must always be ambivalent because of the double example of Christ himself. On the one hand he healed the sick and proclaimed that his miracles were signs of God's great act of redemption. On the other, he allowed himself to be unjustly crucified, suffering hideous agony in the process. At the last supper he taught his disciples by word and act that his death was to be the crux of God's redemptive work; and he warned them that the Christian way was to be a way of the cross.

Sickness, therefore, may provide a 'sign' by its being cured: and it can also provide a convincing 'sign' by its being endured. There have been several remarkable testimonies from cancer victims (of which that quoted in the last chapter is typical) of a new richness of life—for their relatives as well as for themselves—after sentence of death has been passed by their doctors. One such testimony is contained in the book *Margaret*. It is the story of the last three months in the life of a girl of fifteen who died of cancer. The pain of the disease which racked her emaciated body was of no account beside the luminous faith and hope and peace and joy which shone from her spirit and filled her home. It drew from the surgeon who attended her the astonishing comment, 'Margaret was healed, perfectly healed, no matter what state her body was in' (*45*, 151).

At the religious heart of her story lay her confirmation and her regular receiving of Holy Communion. We may well finish our study of healing miracles by a short consideration of the nature of this sacrament, picturesquely described by Ignatius, the martyr-bishop of Antioch early in the second century, as 'the medicine of immortality'. Its nature is essentially miraculous. Its functioning depends upon the power of God, who instituted the sacrament, working through the human agency of his church and through the material products of his creation, bread and wine. It is a non-conforming event which can never be reduced to the descriptive level of the physical sciences. If the consecrated bread and wine are subjected to microscopic examination and chemical analysis, they will be found to be only bread and wine. But such an experiment shows precisely that the essence of the divine disclosure is not amenable to such treatment. The catholic tradition is right to insist that the essence (or 'substance') of the sacrament is other than the essence or 'substance' of bread and wine. The reformed tradition is also right to insist that the sacrament is not just a marvel, but is also a sign making a very special claim about the will and power of God, a claim which must be responded to rightly, worthily, and with faith.

The sacrament of Holy Communion is a sacrament of healing. It brings to a powerful focus the good news of God's self-giving love for a world gone astray; and it also provides the means by which Christians can best make their response and identify themselves with their Lord in his self-giving. In this sacrament people who are too ill to pray can rest upon the continuous intercession of the world-wide Church.

* * * * *

Our study of healing miracles is finished—one dare not say completed. Many will find it unsatisfactory and inconclusive. There is no simple conclusion in matters which deal with the deep things of God and the deep things of man. Our main plea has been to avoid conclusions which are too simple because they ignore those pieces of evidence which are awkward and do not fit easily into an accepted pattern. To talk about God and his activity is to talk in complex terms, at least as complex as the terms 'I' and 'my activity'. If a miracle is an event which discloses the decisive personal activity of God, and if we are to talk of God in personal terms at all, then miracles are not only possible; they are necessary. Here in particular we are given vital clues to the inmost being and purposes of God.

Since God is a living God, the study of miracles is not just an academic exercise. Because we tend to see in this world only what we are looking for, to stay for a while with Moses at the burning bush or with Mary and Martha at the tomb of their brother will help us to sharpen our perception and deepen our understanding of the activity of the Lord the Spirit today and tomorrow.

Bibliography

The literature covering this field is enormous: van der Loos's book alone gives a list of books covering twenty large pages. The following are books and articles which I have consulted and found useful. Several of them contain extensive bibliographies, and these are marked with an asterisk. Unless otherwise stated the books are published in England.

1. *Barrett, C. K., *The Gospel according to St. John*, S.P.C.K., 1955/1956.
2. Bloom, Anthony, *Living Prayer*, Darton, Longman & Todd, 1966.
3. *Bultmann, R., *History of the Synoptic Tradition* (English translation of the 2nd edition), Blackwell, 1921/1931/1963.
4. Caird, G. B., *Saint Luke*, Penguin, 1963.
5. Dodd, C. H., *Historical Tradition in the Fourth Gospel*, C.U.P., 1963.
6. Dunbar, Flanders, *Mind and Body: Psychosomatic Medicine*, Random House (New York), 1947/1966.
7. Fenton, J. C., *Saint Matthew*, Penguin, 1963.
8. Foulkes, S. H. and Anthony, E. J., *Group Psychotherapy*, Penguin, 1957/1965.
9. Frost, Evelyn, *Christian Healing*, Mowbray, 1940.
10. Fuller, R. H., *Interpreting the Miracles*, S.C.M., 1963.
11. Halmos, P., *The Faith of the Counsellors*, Constable, 1965.
12. *Hesse, Mary B., *Science and the Human Imagination*, S.C.M., 1954.
13. James, M. R., *The Apocryphal New Testament*, Oxford, 1924/1945.
14. Johnson, A. R., *The Vitality of the Individual in the Thought of Ancient Israel*, University of Wales Press, 1949/1964.
15. Jones, D. Caradog, *Spiritual Healing*, Longmans, 1955.
16. Kallas, James, *The Significance of the Synoptic Miracles*, S.P.C.K., 1961.
17. Kierkegaard, S., *The Sickness Unto Death*, Doubleday (New York), 1849/1954.
18. *Kissen, D. M., *Emotional Factors in Pulmonary Tuberculosis*, Tavistock, 1958.

19. *Laing, R. D., *The Divided Self*, Penguin, 1959/1965.

20. Lake, Frank, *Clinical Theology*, Darton, Longman & Todd, 1966.

21. *Lambourne, R. A., *Community, Church and Healing*, Darton, Longman & Todd, 1963.

22. *Lawton, J. S., *Miracles and Revelation*, Lutterworth, 1959.

23. Leaney, A. R. C., *A Commentary on the Gospel according to St. Luke*, A. & C. Black, 1958.

24. Lewis, C. S., *Miracles*, Collins, 1947/1964.

25. Locke, John, *The Reasonableness of Christianity* WITH *A Discourse of Miracles*, edited and introduced by I. T. Ramsey, A. & C. Black, 1958.

26. *Loos, H. van der, *The Miracles of Jesus* (Supplement VIIII to *Novum Testamentum*), E. J. Brill (Leiden), 1965.

27. Marshall, Bruce, *Father Malachy's Miracle*, Constable, 1931/1963.

28. Martin, D. V., *Adventure in Psychiatry*, Cassirer, 1962.

29. Martin, D. V., *The Church as a Healing Community*, Guild of Health, n.d.

30. Martin, Denis V., *The Meaning of Faith in Faith-Healing*, Epworth, 1954/1962.

31. Menninger, Karl, *Man Against Himself*, Hart-Davis, 1938.

32. Micklem, E. R., *Miracles and the New Psychology*, O.U.P., 1922.

33. *Monden, Louis, *Le Miracle, Signe de Salut*, Desclée (Bruges), 1960.

34. *Nineham, D. E., *Saint Mark*, Penguin, 1963/1964.

35. *Peursen, C. A. van, *Body, Soul, Spirit: A Survey of the Body–Mind Problem* (English Edition), O.U.P., 1956/1966.

36. Plummer, A., *The Gospel According to St. Luke*, T. & T. Clark, 1896/1905.

37. Rae, J. Burnett, *Chaplain and Doctor*, S.P.C.K., 1949.

38. Ramsey, I. T., *Miracles: An Exercise in Logical Mapwork*, Clarendon, 1952.

39. Ramsey, I. T., *Religion and Science: Conflict and Synthesis*, S.P.C.K., 1964.

40. Raven, Charles E., *Science, Medicine and Morals*, Hodder & Stoughton, 1959.

41. Richardson, A., *The Miracle Stories of the Gospels*, S.C.M., 1941/1963.

42. Robertson, F. W., *Sermons preached at Brighton*, Smith, Elder, 1870.

43. Robinson, James M., *The Problem of History in Mark*, S.C.M., 1957/1962.

44. Robinson, John A. T., *On Being the Church in the World*, S.C.M., 1960.

45. Ross, J. D., *Margaret*, Hodder & Stoughton, 1957.

46. *Rycroft, Charles, *Psychoanalysis Observed*, Constable, 1966.

47. Siirala, Arne, *The Voice of Illness*, Fortress Press (Philadelphia), 1964.

48. Simeons, A. T. W., *Man's Presumptuous Brain: An Evolutionary Interpretation of Psychosomatic Disease*, Dutton (New York), 1961.

49. Stafford-Clark, David, *Psychiatry To-day*, Penguin, 1952/1961.

50. Stengel, E., *Suicide and Attempted Suicide*, Penguin, 1964.

51. *Taylor, Vincent, *The Formation of the Gospel Tradition*, Macmillan, 1933/1945.

52. *Taylor, Vincent, *The Gospel According to St. Mark*, Macmillan, 1952/1957.

53. Tillich, Paul, *The Courage to Be*, Nisbet, 1952/1955.

54. Tillich, Paul, *The New Being*, S.C.M., 1956/1964.

55. Tillich, Paul, *Systematic Theology, Vol. III*, Nisbet, 1964.

56. Tournier, Paul, *The Meaning of Persons*, S.C.M., 1957/1963.

57. Trench, R. C., *Notes on the Miracles of our Lord*, Macmillan, 1884.

58. *Weatherhead, Leslie D., *Psychology, Religion, and Healing*, Hodder & Stoughton, 1951/1963.

59. *Weiss, E. and English, O. S., *Psychosomatic Medicine*, Saunders (Philadelphia), 1943/1960.

60. Wilson, Michael, *The Church is Healing*, S.C.M., 1966.

61. Wolf, S. and Wolff, H. G., *Human Gastric Function*, O.U.P. (New York), 1947.

62. Woods, G. F., *Contemporary Theological Liberalism*, A. & C. Black, 1965.

63. *Young, R. K. and Meiburg, A. L., *Spiritual Therapy*, Hodder & Stoughton, 1961.

COLLECTIONS

64. *Biology and Personality*, edited by I. T. Ramsey, Blackwell, 1965.

65. *The Church's Ministry of Healing* (Report of the Archbishop's Commission), Church Information Office, 1958/1960.

66. *Clergy–Doctor Co-operation*, Church Information Office, 1963.

67. *Decisions about Life and Death*, Church Information Office, 1965.

68. *Divine Healing* (*Nursing Times* reprint), Macmillan, 1959.

69. *Divine Healing and Co-operation between Doctors and Clergy*, British Medical Association, 1956.

70. **The Healing Church*: The Tübingen Consultation 1964, World Council of Churches, 1965.

71. **Health and Community*, 'Study Encounter', Vol. II, No. 3, World Council of Churches, 1966.

72. **Miracles: Cambridge Studies in their Philosophy and History*, edited by C. F. D. Moule, Mowbray, 1965.

73. *Miracles and the Resurrection, The* (Theological Collections No. 3), S.P.C.K., 1964.

74. *Nature of Man, The, in Theological and Psychological Perspective*, edited by Simon Doniger, Harper Bros. (New York), 1962.

75. *New Essays in Philosophical Theology*, edited by Anthony Flew and Alasdair Macintyre, S.C.M., 1955.

76. *Psychophysiological Aspects of Cancer*, edited by E. M. Weyer, New York Academy of Sciences, 1966.

77. *Vindications*: Essays on the Historical Basis of Christianity, edited by Anthony Hanson, S.C.M., 1966.

ARTICLES

78. Bloom, Anthony, 'Suffering', *Church of England Hospital Chaplains' Fellowship*, New Vol. I, No. 1, February 1965.

79. Day, George H., 'From the Sidelines', *Perspectives in Biology and Medicine*, University of Chicago, Winter 1966, Vol. IX, No. 2, pp. 191–207.

80. Joyce, C. R. B., and Welldon, R. M. C. 'The Objective Efficacy of Prayer, a double-blind clinical trial', *Journal of Chronic Diseases*, 1965, Vol. 18, pp. 367–377.

81. Lambourne, R. A., 'What is Healing?', *Frontier*, Spring 1963, Vol. VI, No. 1, pp. 15–18.

82. Lambourne, R. A., 'Judgment in Psychiatry', *Frontier*, Summer 1961, Vol. IV, No. 2, pp. 107–110.

83. Sutherland, John, 'Place of Psychotherapy in Community Mental Health' (and comment by J. A. Whyte), *Contact*, No. 19, January 1967.

84. Taylor, John V., 'Healing and the Gospel', *C.M.S. News-Letter* No. 300, January 1967.

85. Welldon, R. M. C., 'Intercessory Prayer for Healing: Difficulties in Evaluation', Institute of Religion and Medicine, 1967.

Index of Scripture References

A LIST OF HEALING MIRACLE STORIES IN
THE GOSPELS

(in order of treatment)

Index of Subjects and Names

189

ACKNOWLEDGEMENTS

The thanks of the author and publishers are due to the following for permission to quote extracts: E. J. Brill, Leiden, *Miracles of Jesus*, by H. Van der Loos; Bruno Cassirer, *Adventure in Psychiatry* by D. V. Martin; William Heinemann Ltd., *Father and Son* by E. Gosse; Hodder & Stoughton Ltd., *Spiritual Therapy* by R. K. · Young and A. L. Merburg; The New York Academy of Sciences, *Psychophysiological Aspects of Cancer* edited by D. M. Weyer; The University of Chicago Press, *Perspectives in Biology and Medicine*, Winter 1966, Vol. IX, No. 2, from an article entitled 'From the Sidelines' by George H. Day.